Different Aspects of Behçet's Disease

Edited by Müzeyyen Gönül and Arzu Kılıç

Published in London, United Kingdom

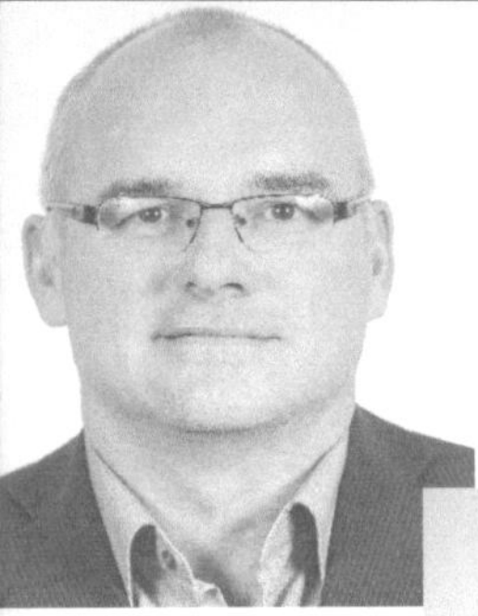
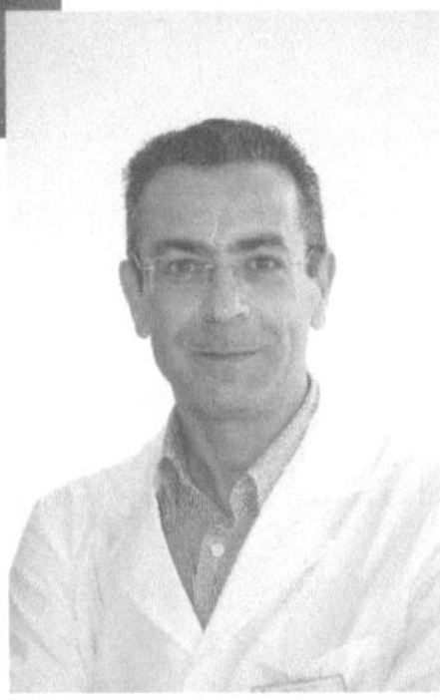
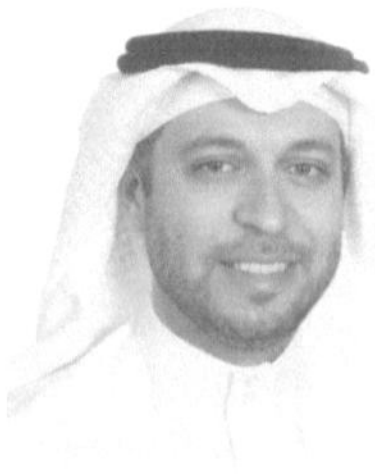
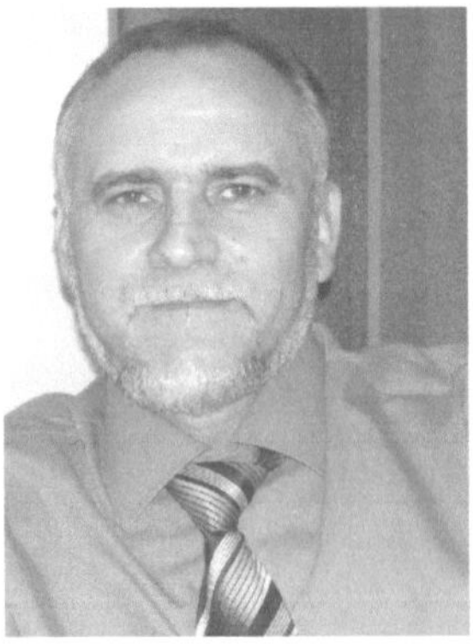
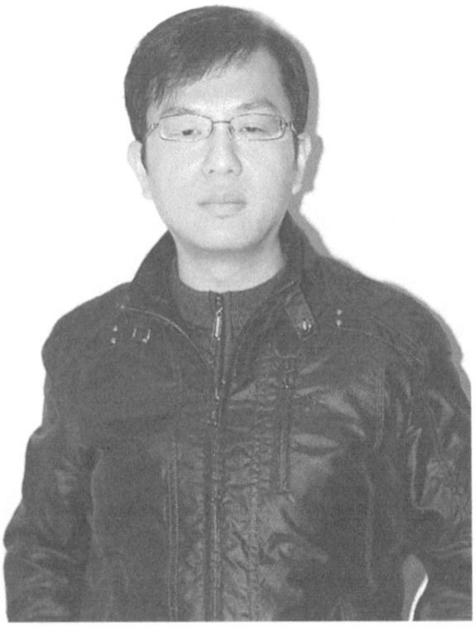
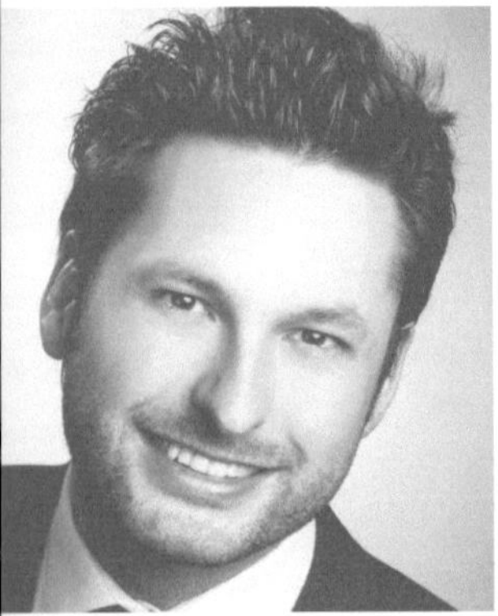
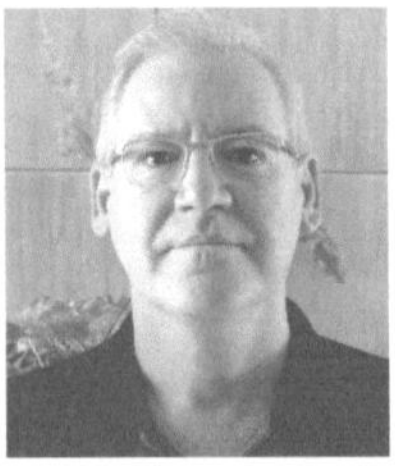

IntechOpen

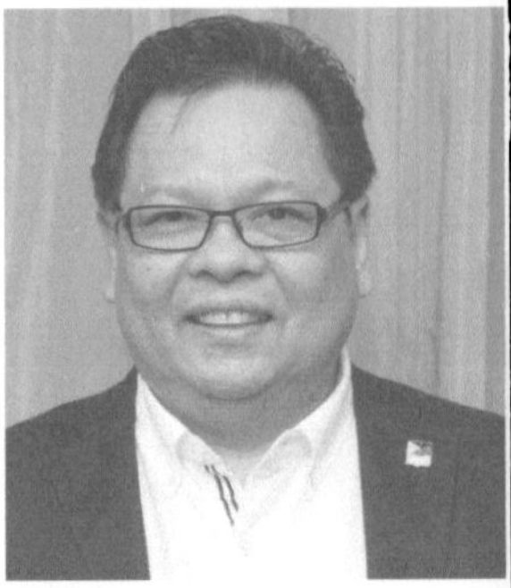
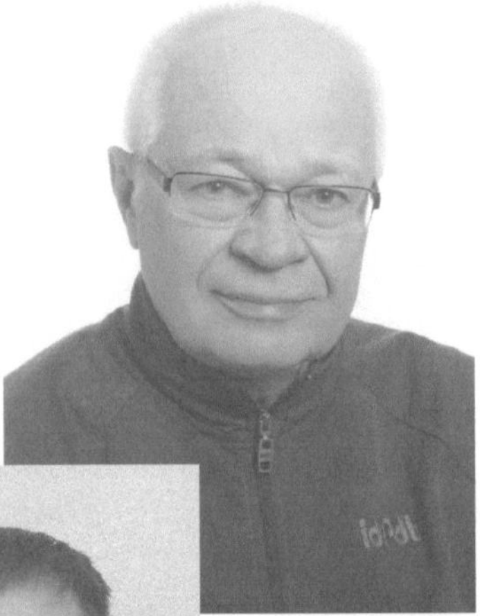
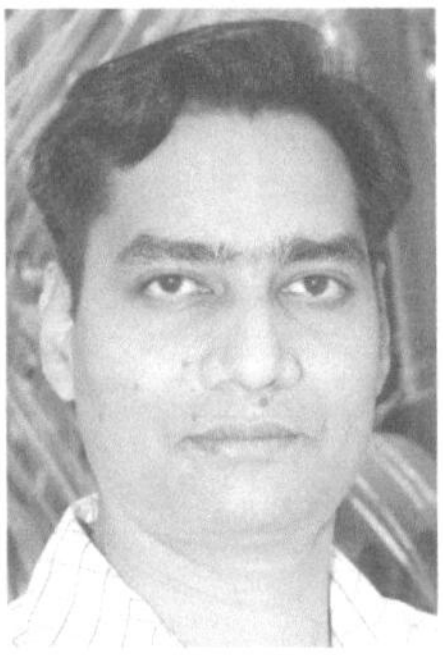
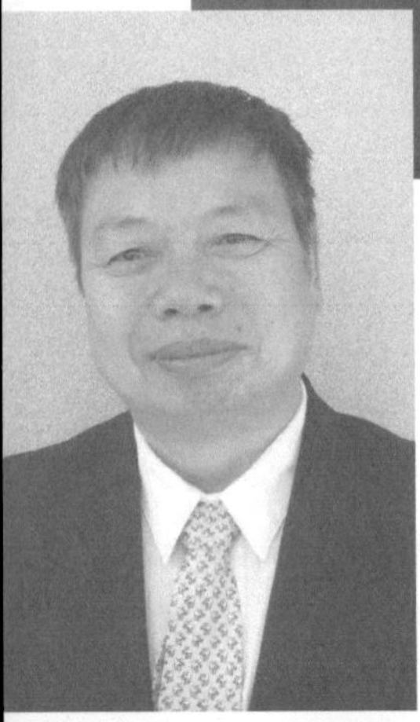
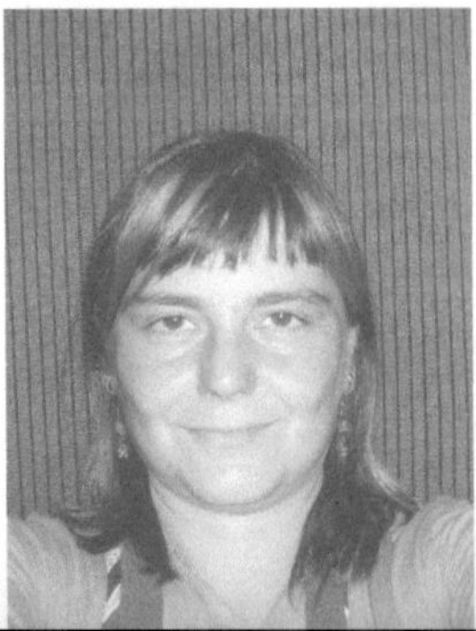
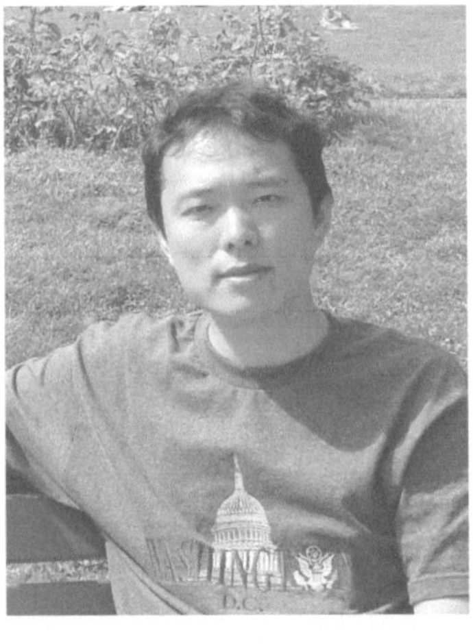

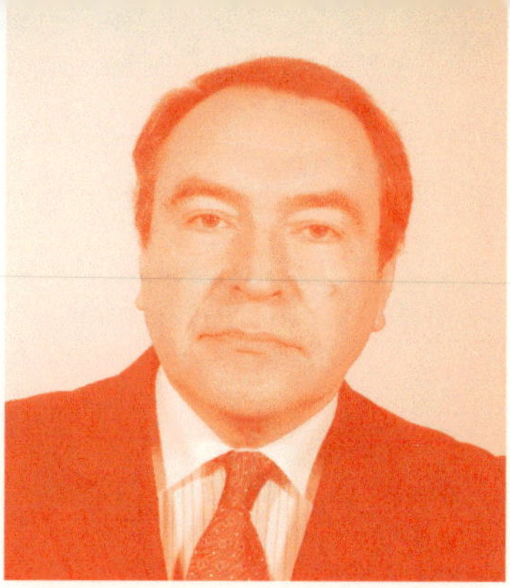
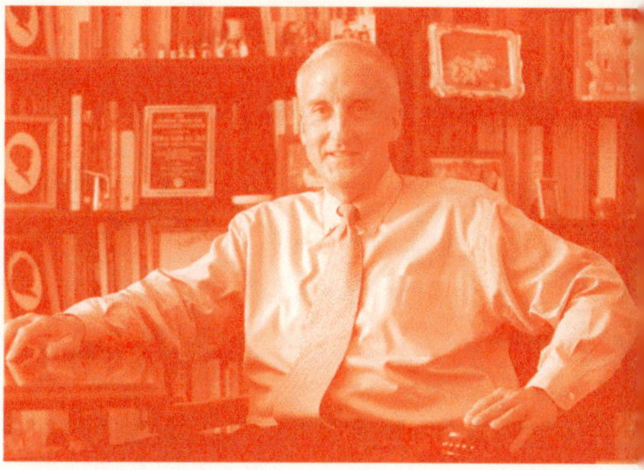
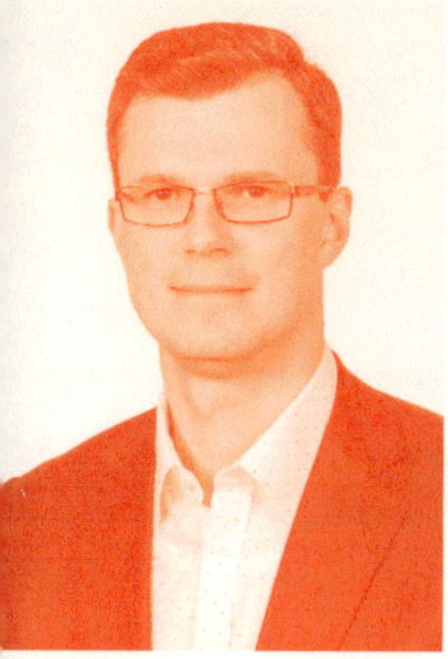
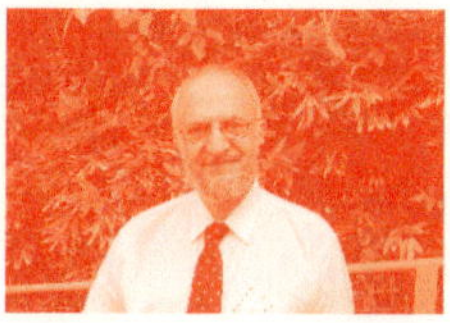
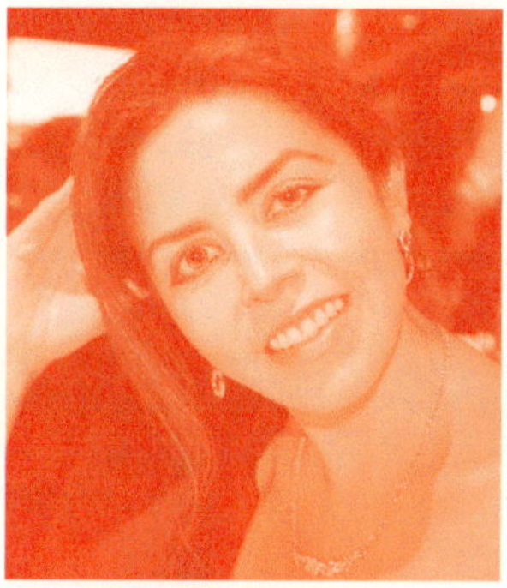

Supporting open minds since 2005

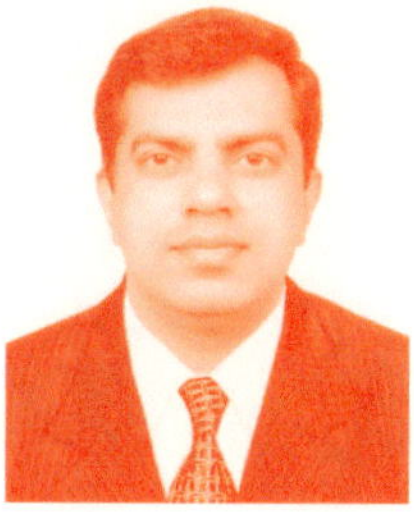
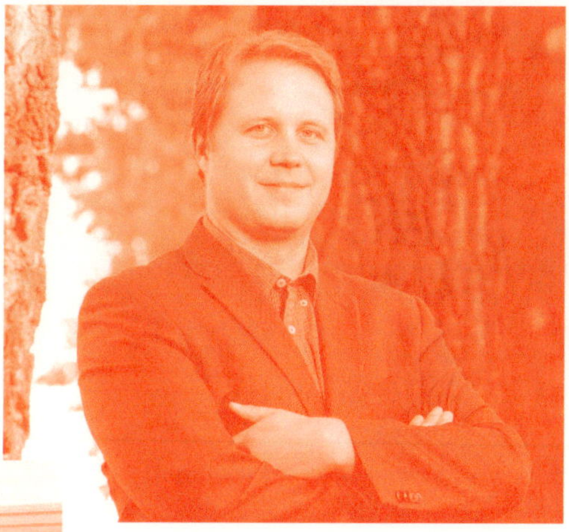
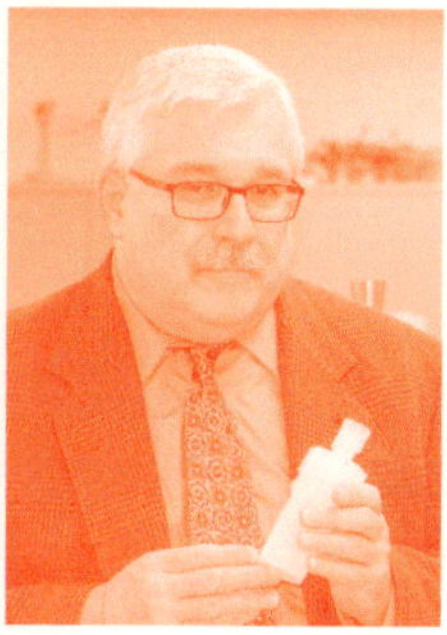
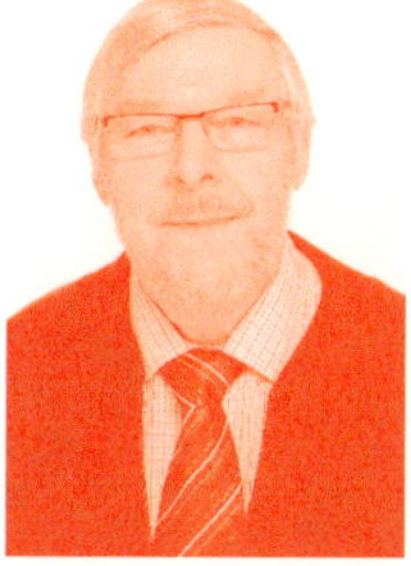
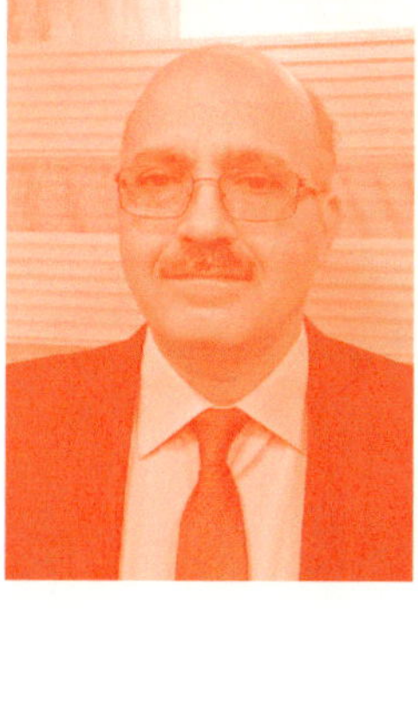
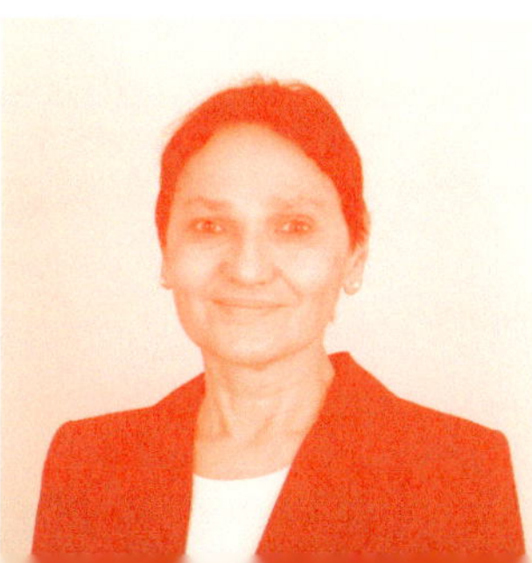
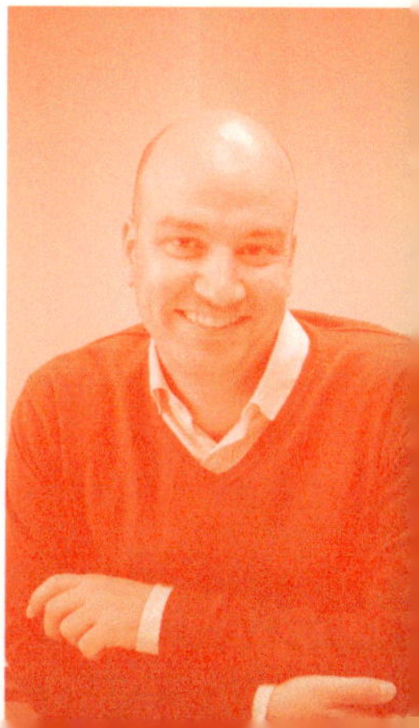

Different Aspects of Behçet's Disease
http://dx.doi.org/10.5772/intechopen.80119
Edited by Müzeyyen Gönül and Arzu Kılıç

Contributors
Xiaodong Zhou, Yan Deng, Shamaz Mohamed, Abhilash R Krishnan, Yuki Nanke, Gökçe Işıl Kurmuş, Erol Koc, Müzeyyen Gönül, Arzu Kılıç, Bilgen Gencler

First published in London, United Kingdom, 2020 by IntechOpen
IntechOpen is the global imprint of INTECHOPEN LIMITED, registered in England and Wales, registration number: 11086078, 7th floor, 10 Lower Thames Street, London, EC3R 6AF, United Kingdom
Printed in Croatia

British Library Cataloguing-in-Publication Data
A catalogue record for this book is available from the British Library

Additional hard and PDF copies can be obtained from orders@intechopen.com

Different Aspects of Behçet's Disease
Edited by Müzeyyen Gönül and Arzu Kılıç
p. cm.
Print ISBN 978-1-78985-659-0
Online ISBN 978-1-78985-660-6
eBook (PDF) ISBN 978-1-78985-992-8

Meet the editors

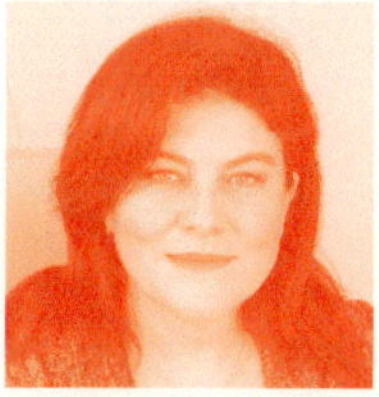

Assoc. Prof. Müzeyyen Gönül graduated from Ankara University School of Medicine. Currently, she is Associate Professor in the Department of Dermatology at the Health Science University, Dışkapı Yıldırım Beyazıt Training and Research Hospital, Ankara, Turkey. She has published approximately 200 articles in international and national journals, three books as editor/co-editor, and six book chapters. Her research interests are psoriasis, urticaria, autoimmune bullous disorders, and Behçet's disease

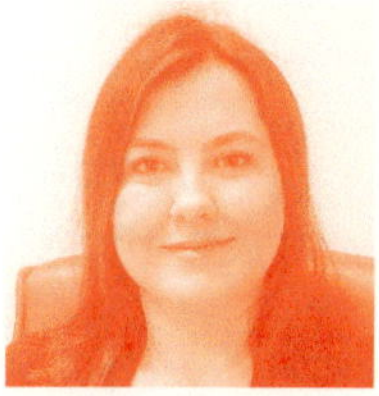

Arzu Kılıç, MD, is the head of the Department of Dermatology at Balikesir University Medical Faculty. She has been working as a professor at the Dermatology Department in Balikesir University School of Medicine, Balikesir, Turkey, since August 2014. She graduated from Gazi University School of Medicine, Ankara, Turkey, in 2000 and worked as a specialist and associate professor in Numune Education and Research Hospital, Ankara, Turkey, between 2004 and 2014. Dr. Kılıç has published several articles in more than 80 international, peer-reviewed ISI-JCR journals and more than 60 national journals. She has also published three book chapters and more than 50 conference proceedings. She has also edited one book and has supervised several medical students.

Contents

Preface

Behçet's disease is a chronic, relapsing, inflammatory multisystem disease characterized by oral and genital ulcers, cutaneous lesions, and ocular and articular involvement of unknown etiology. It can also affect the gastrointestinal, cardiovascular, and nervous systems. It can cause severe systemic involvement, morbidity, and even mortality. Genetic factors have been investigated extensively, and have defined new genetic polimorphisms associated with the disease. Research into the immunopathogenesis of Behçet's disease has increased our knowledge of this subject. The diagnosis of Behçet's disease is based on clinical criteria, as there is no pathognomonic test. In Behçet disease, there is a wide variety of mucocutaneous and systemic findings that can be confused with many diseases in differential diagnosis. Therefore, being aware of the disease and recognizing the mucocutaneous symptoms would lead to accurate diagnosis. The aim of this book is to present information to our colleagues in different branches of medicine by discussing the genetic and immunologic etiopathogenesis, clinical features, and relationship with pregnancy of Behçet's disease in five chapters:

- The history and diagnosis of Behçet's disease
- Behçet's disease: an enigmatic malady with plethoric expressions
- Genetics of Behçet's disease
- The role of Th17 cells in the pathogenesis of Behçet's disease
- Behçet's disease and pregnancy

We believe that this book will be a valuable reference to students, researchers, dermatologists, and other healthcare professionals interested in Behçet's disease. We are very grateful to all the authors for their efforts and patience needed to bring about this book.

Müzeyyen Gönül, MD
Associate Professor,
Health Science University,
Dışkapı Yıldırım Beyazıt Training and Research Hospital
Dermatology Clinic,
Ankara, Turkey

Arzu Kılıç, MD
Professor,
Balıkesir University,
Dermatology Department,
Balıkesir, Turkey

Section 1

An Overview of Behçet's Disease

Chapter 1

The History and Diagnosis of Behçet's Disease

Müzeyyen Gönül, Arzu Kılıç and Bilgen Gençler

Abstract

Behçet's disease (BD) is a multisystemic vasculitis of unknown aetiology, initially reported by Turkish dermatologist Hulusi Behçet in 1937. Hulusi Behçet presented the disease as a triple symptom complex with recurrent aphthosis, genital ulceration and recurrent hypopyon uveitis. But subsequent studies have shown that it can affect many organs with wide clinical spectrum. It is challenging to make a definite diagnosis because there is no pathognomic laboratory test to diagnose Behçet's disease. The diagnosis is based on variable group of clinical manifestations. Many new diagnostic/classification criteria have been developed through the years. International Study Group (ISG) Criteria and the International Criteria for Behçet's Disease (ICBD) are the most commonly acceptable criteria for the diagnosis of BD. However, due to the broad clinical spectrum of Behçet's disease, there will always be Behçet's patients who do not complete the criteria. Therefore, the experience of the physician and evaluation of the findings with a good clinical anamnesis is of great importance in the diagnosis.

Keywords: Hulusi Behçet, Behçet's disease, International Study Group criteria, International Criteria for Behçet's disease

1. Introduction

Behçet's disease (BD) is a multisystemic vasculitis according to the 2012 Revised International Chapel Hill Consensus Conference Nomenclature of Vasculitides [1]. The autoimmune process, which is triggered by the environmental and infectious factors on the basis of the genetic factors, is held responsible for the formation of the disease [2]. The definition of the disease dates back to ancient times until the time of Hippocrates [3]. However, for the first time in modern medicine in 1937, Prof. Dr. Hulusi Behçet described it as a separate entity consisting of oral aphthosis, genital ulceration, and iridocyclitis with hypopyon [4].

2. Hulusi Behçet: a life dedicated to dermatology (the person behind the eponym)

Hulusi Behçet was born on 20 February 1889 in Istanbul. Hulusi Behçet was raised by his grandmother after his mother's death when he was young and he had a difficult childhood. He settled in Damascus because of his father's work. He studied at a French school and learned French, Latin, and German. In 1906, he started Kuleli Military Medical School when he was only 16 years old and graduated in 1910.

After his specialization training on skin and venereal diseases in Gulhane Military Hospital, he worked in Edirne Military hospital for 4 years. Afterwards, he went to Europe and worked in Budapest and Berlin for a short time and returned to his country. He worked as a freelance doctor for a while, and then he worked at Haskoy Venereal Diseases Hospital and Guraba Hospital after that in 1933; he became the head of the Department of Skin and Venereal Diseases of Istanbul University and continued this position until 1947 [5, 6].

He is interested in many different areas of dermatology such as syphilis, leishmaniasis, dermatitis *Figus carcia*, parasitosis, and mycosis, but he is mostly known for his studies on Behçet's disease, which is named after him. He presented his research in many national and international meetings and congresses and published 126 articles between 1921 and 1940 [5, 6].

Studies on Behçet's disease began with a patient he first saw in 1924.The patient had recurrent hypopyon uveitis accompanied by ulcerations in the mouth and scrotum, painful nodules on the legs, fever, and joint pain and was variously diagnosed in Istanbul and Vienna and was followed by Hulusi Behçet later on for many more years [5–7].

In 1930, he conducted a study on a female patient with recurrent ocular symptoms and oral and genital lesions and in 1936 on a male patient with oral pemphigus-like wounds, acneiform lesions on the back, scrotal ulcer, night fever, abdominal pain, and ocular symptoms [5–7].

As a result of his research on these three patients, Hulusi Behçet first suggested in 1937 that recurrent oral aphthous lesions, genital ulceration, and recurrent hypopyon uveitis were the symptoms of a single disease as a triple symptom complex [4]. He wrote this view in 1937 in the journal *Dermatologische Wochenschrift* and presented it to his colleagues at a congress in France in the same year. At the same congress, it was suggested that viruses may play a role in the etiology of this condition, especially those of dental origin [5, 6, 8] (**Figure 1**).

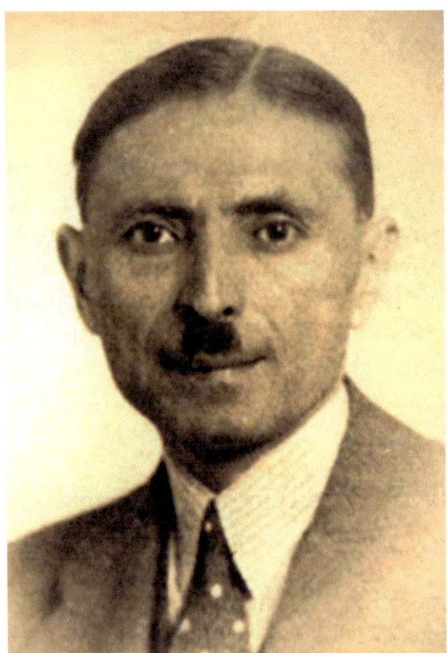

Figure 1.
Hulusi Behçet MD (1889–1948).

In 1938, *Dermatologische Wohenschrift* published his thoughts in more detail. In the following years, new case reports came from different countries. While ophthalmologists accepted this new disease, dermatologists believed it to be a symptom of another existing skin disease. However, as a result of the new articles published in different parts of the world, the disease was accepted to be a separate entity. At the international medical congress in Geneva, with the suggestion of Prof. Mischner from Zurich Medical Faculty, this newly diagnosed disease was called "Morbus Behçet" [5, 6].

In 1930, Dr. Benedictos Adamantiades (1875–1962), a Greek ophthalmologist, reported a patient with recurrent hypopyonic irritation accompanied by mucocutaneous lesions and arthritis [9]. In later years, he wrote new case reports, but he did not interpret this as a triple complex; focusing only on the eye, he suggested that hypopyonic iridocyclitis was a separate clinical disease by itself [10–12]. Undoubtedly, although his colleagues from many parts of the world contributed to the acceptance of Behçet's disease as a separate clinical entity, the first person to describe the triple triad and to present it to the world through his articles and presentations is our esteemed professor, doctor Hulusi Behçet.

3. The diagnosis and classification criteria of Behçet's disease

Firstly, although Behçet's disease is accepted as a triple symptom complex with recurrent aphthosis, genital ulceration, and recurrent hypopyon uveitis, subsequent studies have shown that it is a multisystemic chronic inflammatory disease that can affect many organs [1, 13].

There is no pathognomic laboratory test to diagnose Behçet's disease. The disease's wide clinical spectrum, its showing ethnical and geographical differences, and the differences that it shows in the time of onset of symptoms and its courses with different findings in each patient are the factors that make it difficult to diagnose. Therefore, the experience of the physician and evaluation of the findings with a good clinical anamnesis is of great importance in the diagnosis [14].

Although it is a relatively young disease, many different diagnostic/classification criteria have been developed. The first one was created by Curth in 1946 [15]. In 1969, Hewitt et al. presented the diagnostic criteria and revised and reformed them in 1971 [16, 17]. Many new diagnostic criteria have been established in the light of the studies that have been carried out until today. The main ones are Mason and Barnes in 1969, Japan criteria in 1972, Hubault and Hamza in 1974, O'Duffy in 1974, Chen in 1980, Dilsen et al. in 1986, Japan revised criteria in 1988, International Study Group (ISG) in 1990, Iran in 1993, Classification Tree in 1993, Dilsen revised in 2000, Korea in 2003, the International Criteria for Behçet's Disease (ICBD) in 2006, and the revised ICBD in 2014 [18–32].

The Japan Research Committee for Behçet's Disease created the Japanese criteria in 1972. There are four major symptoms according to these criteria: oral aphthosis, genital aphthosis, skin lesions, and ocular findings. In the presence of an ocular lesion, one different major finding is sufficient for the diagnosis. If there are no ocular findings, the presence of the other three major findings is essential for the diagnosis. It is called "complete form" if there are four major findings, and it is called "incomplete form" if there are fewer findings [19]. Japan criteria were revised in 1988. Five minor findings were added to the major findings, and two minor findings were suggested to replace one missing major finding. These minor findings include arthritis/arthralgia, gastrointestinal manifestations, vascular thrombosis, neurological manifestations, and epididymitis [24].

In the Fourth International Conference on Behçet's Disease, which was held in London in 1985, it was planned to establish a diagnostic criterion with high sensitivity and specificity. Therefore, the International Behçet's Disease Study Group was established [25, 33]. In 7 countries (France, Iran, Japan, Tunisia, Turkey, the UK, and the USA) and in 12 separate institutions, 912 Behçet patients together with 308 control patients were included in a study and followed up. Twenty-eight patients without oral ulceration were excluded from the study [25]. In the light of the data obtained, "International Behçet's Disease Study Group Classification Criteria" was established and published in 1990. ISG classification criteria consist of five items. The first criterion is recurrent oral ulceration at least three times a year and is a sine qua non. The other four criteria consist of recurrent genital ulceration, eye lesions (anterior uveitis, posterior uveitis, retinal vasculitis), skin lesions (erythema nodosum, pseudofolliculitis, or papulopustular lesions), and positive pathergy test. In addition to the major criterion oral aphthosis, the existence of two of the four findings is enough for the diagnosis of Behçet's disease [25, 34] (**Table 1**).

The sensitivity and specificity of ISG classification criteria were found to be 92 and 97%, respectively [25]. Although it is one of the most widely used criteria to date, several concerns about its sensitivity have arisen. In fact, many studies have been performed that measure the performance of diagnostic/classification criteria for Behçet's disease. Because of the high specificity of ISG, the risk of another disease being misdiagnosed and classified as BD is very low. However, many Behçet's disease patients go undiagnosed due to its low sensitivity [35]. Another controversial issue is that oral aphthosis is an indispensable finding in ISG, but it has been shown that oral aphthosis may not be in 1–10% of BD patients [36]. Behçet patients with severe, specific symptoms such as vascular involvement can also go without diagnosis with these criteria, and thus the concern of delay in treatment has arisen [37, 38].

In 1993, Iran presented the ISG criteria in an international conference by modifying them to overcome the problem of low sensitivity and low accuracy. According to these criteria, it consisted of five items similar to ISG, but oral aphthosis was not mandatory. Oral aphthosis was given 2 points, and other lesions were given 1 point, and 3 points were sufficient to diagnose BD [26].

In 1993, Iran released a new classification system, using the Classification and Regression Tree method, called the classification tree. The presence of one of the five subgroups in the patient alone is sufficient to diagnose BD. These subgroups are as follows: oral aphthosis + genital aphthosis, oral aphthosis + skin lesions + positive

Recurrent oral ulceration	Minor or major aphthous ulceration or herpetiform ulceration observed by physician or patient (at least three occurrences within a 12-month period)
Plus any two of the following criteria	
Recurrent genital ulceration	Aphthous ulceration or scarring observed by the physician or patient
Eye lesions	Anterior uveitis, posterior uveitis, or cells in vitreous on slit-lamp examination or retinal vasculitis detected by an ophthalmologist
Skin lesions	Erythema nodosum observed by physician or patient, pseudofolliculitis, or papulopustular lesions or acneiform nodules observed by the physician in postadolescent patients (not receiving corticosteroid treatment)
Positive pathergy test	Read by physician at 24–48 hours.

Findings applicable only in the absence of other clinical explanations.

Table 1.
International study group (ISG) criteria for the diagnosis of Behçet's disease.

pathergy test, oral aphthosis + ocular findings, genital aphthosis + ocular findings, and positive pathergy test + ocular findings [27].

In 2000, the original criteria were revised by Dilsen, suggesting that three of the six diagnostic criteria were sufficient to diagnose BD. These criteria are oral aphthosis, genital ulceration, skin lesions (pseudofolliculitis, erythema nodosum), ocular findings, thrombophlebitis, and positive pathergy test [28].

In 2003, Korea established its own diagnostic criterion for BD. This criterion contains six items: oral aphthosis, genital ulceration, skin lesions, ocular findings, positive pathergy test, and gastrointestinal involvement. Three points and above is sufficient to diagnose BD with three points for genital ulceration and one point for other findings [29].

In 2003 the First International Workshop of Behçet's Disease was held in Austria. In this workshop, it was decided that a team of eight countries would prepare a proposal to develop the ISG criteria and to establish new criteria for Behçet's disease if necessary [35].

In the 11th International Conference on Behçet's Disease in Antalya (Turkey) in 2004, the International Team for the Revision of the ISG criteria was created which was composed of clinicians from 27 countries. Among these countries, in the first place comes Turkey, and the rest were Austria, Azerbaijan, China, Egypt, France, Germany, Greece, India, Iran, Iraq, Israel, Italy, Japan, Jordan, Libya, Morocco, Pakistan, Portugal, Russia, Saudi Arabia, Singapore, Spain, Taiwan, Thailand, Tunisia, and the USA.

Between January 2005 and June 2006, 2556 BD and 1163 control patients were included in a study who were selected by expert opinion, rather than a classification system. The International Criteria for Behçet's Disease included a new scoring system for the diagnosis of Behçet's disease. It consisted of six items: genital ulceration and ocular findings with 2 points and oral aphthosis, skin lesions, vascular lesions, and pathergy test with 1 point. A score of 3 or more was sufficient for the diagnosis of BD. In 2010, ICBD criteria were revised and presented at the 14th International Conference on Behçet's Disease in London. In 2014, these criteria were published in the *Journal of the European Academy of Dermatology and Venereology*. The differences from the classical form were the addition of neurological findings as 1 point and the increase of oral aphthosis to 2 points. Pathergy test was optional but 1 point should be added at its presence. Four points and above was sufficient for the diagnosis of Behçet's disease. The sensitivity and specificity of ICBD was 94.8 and 90.5%, respectively [30–32] (**Table 2**).

Sign/symptom points	
Oral aphthosis	2
Genital ulceration	2
Ocular lesions	2
Skin lesions	1
Vascular manifestations	1
Neurological manifestations	1
Positive pathergy test*	1

**1-Pathergy test is optional. However, when it is performed, one extra point may be assigned for a positive result.*
2-A patient scoring 4 points or above was classified as having Behçet's disease.

Table 2.
The international criteria for Behçet's disease (ICBD)—point-score system.

4. Differential diagnosis of Behçet's disease

Since Behçet's disease has a broad clinical spectrum, many diseases are included in the differential diagnosis. Although many diagnostic criteria have been developed, it can still be difficult to diagnose Behçet's disease, and it may be necessary to exclude diseases that show similar findings in the differential diagnosis.

4.1 Differential diagnosis of mucocutaneous findings

4.1.1 Oral aphthosis

Recurrent aphthous stomatitis (RAS), viral infections such as herpes simplex virus and Coxsackievirus infections, nutritional deficiencies such as vitamin B and iron, recurrent erythema multiform, oral erosive lichen planus, autoimmune bullous diseases, fixed drug eruption, Stevens-Johnson syndrome, toxic epidermal necrolysis, inflammatory bowel diseases (IBD), Reiter syndrome, systemic lupus erythematosus, celiac disease, mouth and genital ulcers with inflamed cartilage (MAGIC) syndrome, must be Periodic Fever, Aphthous Stomatitis, Pharyngitis, Adenitis (PFAPA) syndrome, hematologic malignancies, and trauma [39–42].

4.1.2 Genital ulceration

Herpes simplex infection; erosive lichen planus; autoimmune bullous dermatoses; sexually transmitted infectious diseases, especially syphilis; and fixed drug eruption [41, 43].

4.1.3 Skin lesions

Papulopustular lesions can be confused with acne and bacterial folliculitis [14, 44].

4.2 Differential diagnosis of systemic findings

The diseases of the similar systemic findings with BD are inflammatory bowel diseases, seronegative arthropathies, sarcoidosis, lupus erythematosus and other systemic vasculitis, multiple sclerosis as neurological involvement, and stroke of the young adult [14, 45].

Differential diagnosis of BD from IBD may be challenging for clinicians because findings of both two diseases include gastrointestinal manifestations, fever, oral aphthosis, pyoderma gangrenosum, erythema nodosum, Sweet syndrome like dermatosis, neutrophilic lobular panniculitis, ocular involvement, arthritis, vasculitis, and thrombotic events. Moreover, the manifestations of intestinal BD are similar to IBD. There are no diagnostic laboratory tests or endoscopic findings for the differential diagnosis of both diseases. Endoscopic findings of Behçet's disease demonstrate single or few, large, round, or oval-shaped ulcerations. Longitudinal ulcers in a discontinuous distribution and cobblestone appearance are endoscopic features of IBD. However, neurologic involvement is not observed in IBD [46–50].

Bowel-associated dermatosis-arthritis syndrome (BADAS) is a recurrent neutrophilic dermatosis which is associated with bowel bypass surgery and gastrointestinal disorders like IBD and diverticulitis [51, 52]. The syndrome should be distinguished from BD, due to the similar findings such as oral aphthosis, vesiculopustular dermatosis, erythema nodosum, neutrophilic lobular panniculitis, fever, vasculitis, and arthritis. The other cutaneous findings of BD and ocular and neurologic involvement are not expected findings for BADAS. The pathergy test is also negative in the BADAS patients [50].

Although many criteria have been developed for the diagnosis of Behçet's disease, there are still a number of difficulties to establish a definitive diagnosis and for making differential diagnosis. Therefore, newly defined molecular markers and universal criteria with high sensitivity and specificity are needed.

Author details

Müzeyyen Gönül[1]*, Arzu Kılıç[2] and Bilgen Gençler[1]

1 Dermatology Clinic, University of Health Sciences, Dışkapı Yıldırım Beyazıt Education and Research Hospital, Turkey

2 Dermatology Department, Balıkesir University, Turkey

*Address all correspondence to: muzeyyengonul@gmail.com

References

[1] Davatchi F, Chams-Davatchi C, Shams H, Shahram F, Nadji A, Akhlaghi M, et al. Behçet's disease: Epidemiology, clinical manifestations, and diagnosis. Expert Review of Clinical Immunology. 2017;**13**(1):57-65

[2] Greco A, De Virgilio A, Ralli M, Ciofalo A, Mancini P, Attanasio G, et al. Behçet's disease: New insights into pathophysiology, clinical features and treatment options. Autoimmunity Reviews. 2018;**17**(6):567-575

[3] Feigenbaum A. Description of Behçet's syndrome in the hippocratic third book of endemic diseases. The British Journal of Ophthalmology. 1956;**40**:355-357

[4] Behçet H. Uber rezidivierende aphthosa, durch ein Virus verüsachte Geschewüre am Mund, am Auge und an den Genitalien. Dermatologische Wochenschrift. 1937;**109**:1152-1157

[5] Saylan T. Life story of Dr. Hulusi Behçet. Yonsei Medical Journal. 1997;**38**(6):327-332

[6] Tüzün Y. Hulusi Behçet MD: February 20, 1889 to March 8, 1948. Clinics in Dermatology. 2006;**24**(6):548-550

[7] Evereklioglu C. Behçet's disease or Adamantiades-Behçet disease? An evidence-based historical survey. Medical Science Monitor. 2010;**16**(6):136-142

[8] Behçet H, Gözcü N. Üç Nahiyede Nüksi Tavazzular Yapan ve Hususi Bir Virus Tesiri ile Umumi İntan Hasıl Ettiğine Kanaatimiz Artan Entite Morbide Hakkında. Deri Hastalıkları ve Frengi Kliniği Arşivi. 1938;**5**:1863-1873

[9] Adamantiades B. A case of recurrent hypopyon iritis. Proceedings of the Medical Society of Athens. 1930:586-593

[10] Adamantiades B. La thrombophlébite comme quatrième symptôme de l'iritis récidivante à hypopyon. The Annales d'Oculistique et de Gynecologie (Paris). 1946;**179**:143-148

[11] Adamantiades B. Le symptôme complexe de l'uvéite récidivante à hypopyon (the complex syndrome of recurrent uveitis with hypopyon). The Annales d'Oculistique et de Gynecologie (Paris). 1953;**186**(9):846-856

[12] Adamantiades B. Severe complications of the central nervous system in the syndrome of relapsing iritis with hypopyon (in Greek). Deltion Ellikinis Ophthalmologikis Etairias. 1958;**26**:199-202

[13] Alpsoy E. Behçet's disease: A comprehensive review with a focus on epidemiology, etiology and clinical features, and management of mucocutaneous lesions. The Journal of Dermatology. 2016;**43**(6):620-632

[14] Boyvat A. Behçet Hastalığında Tanı ve Ayırıcı Tanı. Turkiye Klinikleri Dermatology-Special Topics. 2017;**10**(4):315-320

[15] Curth HO. Recurrent genito-oral aphthosis with hypopion (Behçet's syndrome). Archives of Dermatology;**54**:179-196

[16] Hewitt J, Escande JP, Laurent PH, Perlemuter L. Criteres de prevision du syndrome de Behçet. Bulletin de la SocieteFrancaise de Dermatology et de Syphiligraphie. 1969;**76**:565-568

[17] Hewitt J, Escande JP, Manesse S. Revision of the diagnostic criteria of Behçet's syndrome. La Presse Médicale. 1971;**79**:901

[18] Mason RM, Barnes CG. Behçet's syndrome with arthritis. The Annals of the Rheumatic Diseases;**28**:95-103

[19] Behçet's Disease Research Committee of Japan. Behçet's disease guide to the diagnosis of Behçet's disease (1972). Japanese Journal of Ophthalmology. 1974;**18**:291-294

[20] Hubault A, Hamza M. La maladie de Behçet en 1974. In: de Sezeet S et al., editors. L'actualit'e Rhumatologique 15. Paris, France: Expension Scientifique; 1974. pp. 43-55

[21] O'Duffy JD. Crit'eres propos'es pour le diagnostique de la maladie de Behçet et notes therapeutiques. Revista Médica. 1974;**36**:2371-2379

[22] Cheng SP, Zhang X-Q. Some special clinical manifestations of Behçet's disease—Report of illustrative cases and review of literature (author's transl). The Chinese Journal of Internal Medicine;**19**:15-22

[23] Dilsen N, Konice M, Aral O. Our diagnostic criteria of Behçet's disease—An overview. In: Lehner T, Barnes CG, editor. Recent Advances in Behçet's Disease. Vol. 103. International Congress and Symposium Series. London, UK: London Royal Society of Medicine Services; 1986. pp. 177-180

[24] Mizushima Y. Recent research into Behçet's disease in Japan. International Journal of Tissue Reactions. 1988;**10**:59-65

[25] International Study Group for Behçet's Disease. Criteria for diagnosis of Behçet's disease. Lancet. 1990;**335**(8697):1078-1080

[26] Davatchi F, Shahram F, Akbarian M, et al. Accuracy of existing diagnosis criteria for Behçet's disease. In: Wechsler B, Godeau P, editors. Behçet's Disease. Vol. 1037. Amsterdam, The Netherlands: Excerpta Medica International Congress Series; 1993. pp. 225-228

[27] Davatchi F, Shahram F, Akbarian M, et al. Classification tree for the diagnosis of Behçet's disease. In: Wechsler B, Godeau P, editors. Behçet's Disease. Vol. 1037. Amsterdam, The Netherlands: Excerpta Medica International Congress Series; 1993. pp. 245-248

[28] Dilsen N. About diagnostic criteria for Behçet's disease: Our new proposal. In: Bang D, Lee ES, Lee S, editors. Behçet's Disease. Seoul, Korea: Design Mecca Publishing; 2000. pp. 101-104

[29] Chang HK, Kim SY. Survey and validation of the criteria for Behçet's disease recently used in Korea: A suggestion for modification of the international study group criteria. Journal of Korean Medical Science;**18**:88-92

[30] International Team for the Revision of the International Criteria for Behçet's Disease. Evaluation of the international criteria for Behçet's disease (ICBD). Clinical and Experimental Rheumatology. 2006;**24**(42):13

[31] International Team for the Revision of the International Criteria for Behçet's disease. Revision of the international criteria for Behçet's disease (ICBD). Clinical and Experimental Rheumatology. 2006;**24**(42):14-15

[32] International Team for the Revision of the International Criteria for Behçet's disease (ITR-ICBD), Davatchi F, Assaad-Khalil S, Calamia KT, et al. The International Criteria for Behçet's Disease (ICBD): A collaborative study of 27 countries on the sensitivity and specificity of the new criteria. Journal of the European Academy of Dermatology and Venereology. 2014, 2014;**28**:338-347

[33] Evaluation of Diagnostic (Classification) Criteria in Behçet's

Disease: Toward Internationally Agreed Criteria. International Study Group for Behçet's Disease. In: O'Duffy JD, Komken E, editors. Behçet's Disease. Papers Presented at the Fifth International Conference on Behçet's Disease. New York: Marcel Dekker Inc; 1991. pp. 11-39

[34] Wechsler B, Davatchi F, Mizushima Y, Hamza M, Dilsen N, Kansu E, et al. International Study Group for Behçet's Disease. Evaluation of diagnostic ('classification') criteria in Behçet's disease-toward internationally agreed criteria. British Journal of Rheumatology. 1992;**31**:299-308

[35] Davatchi F, Sadeghi Abdollahi B, Chams-Davatchi C, Shahram F, Shams H, Nadji A, et al. The saga of diagnostic/classification criteria in Behçet's disease. International Journal of Rheumatic Diseases. 2015;**18**(6):594-605

[36] Davatchi F, Shahram F, Chams-Davatchi C, et al. Behçet's disease: From east to west. Clinical Rheumatology. 2010;**29**:823-833

[37] Mignogna MD, Fedele S, Lo Russo L. International diagnostic criteria and delay of diagnosis in Behçet's disease. The Journal of Rheumatology. 2000;**27**(11):2725

[38] Dilsen N. The importance of the manifestations besides the ones included in international criteria for Behçet's disease. Advances in Experimental Medicine and Biology. 2003;**528**:105-108

[39] Muñoz-Corcuera M, Esparza-Gómez G, González-Moles MA, Bascones-Martínez A. Oral ulcers: Clinical aspects. A tool for dermatologists. Part I. Acute ulcers. Clinical and Experimental Dermatology. 2009;**34**(3):289-294

[40] Femiano F, Lanza A, Buonaiuto C, Gombos F, Cirillo N. Oral aphthous-like lesions, PFAPA syndrome: A review. Journal of Oral Pathology and Medicine. 2008;**37**(6):319-323

[41] Köse O. Behçet hastalığında tanı ve ayırıcı tanı. Türkderm. 2009;**43** (Suppl 2):87-91

[42] Talacko AA, Gordon AK, Aldred MJ. The patient with recurrent oral ulceration. Australian Dental Journal. 2010;**55**(Suppl 1):14-22

[43] Roett MA, Mayor MT, Uduhiri KA. Diagnosis and management of genital ulcers. American Family Physician. 2012;**85**(3):254-262

[44] Kalkan G, Karadag AS, Astarci HM, Akbay G, Ustun H, Eksioglu M. A histopathological approach: When papulopustular lesions should be in the diagnostic criteria of Behçet's disease? Journal of the European Academy of Dermatology and Venereology. 2009;**23**(9):1056-1060

[45] Siva A, Altintas A, Saip S. Behçet's syndrome and the nervous system. Current Opinion in Neurology. 2004;**17**(3):347-357

[46] Baptista B, Marto N, Tavares JG, Horta AB, Cunha E Sá D, Gerardo G, et al. Behçet syndrome and Crohn's disease: What are the differences? The European Journal of Case Reports in Internal Medicine. 2019;**6**(3)

[47] Ye JF, Guan JL. Differentiation between intestinal Behçet's disease and Crohn's disease based on endoscopy. Turkish Journal of Medical Sciences. 2019;**49**(1):42-49

[48] Jung YS, Cheon JH, Park SJ, Hong SP, Kim TI, Kim WH. Long-term clinical outcomes of Crohn's disease and intestinal Behçet's disease. Inflammatory Bowel Diseases. 2013;**19**(1):99-105

[49] Valenti S, Gallizzi R, De Vivo D, Romano C. Intestinal Behçet

and Crohn's disease: Two sides of the same coin. Pediatric Rheumatology Online Journal. 2017;**15**(1):33

[50] Davis MDP, Moschella SL. Behçet's syndrome. In: Bolognia JL, Schaffer JV, Cerroni L, editors. Dermatology. 4th ed. Philadelphia: Elsevier; 2017. pp. 463-466

[51] Oldfield CW, Heffernan-Stroud LA, Buehler-Bota TS, Williams JV. Bowel-associated dermatosis-arthritis syndrome (BADAS) in a pediatric patient. JAAD Case Reports. 2016;**2**(3):272-274

[52] Truchuelo MT, Acantara J, Vano-Galvan S, Jaen P. Bowel-associated dermatosis-arthritis syndrome: Another cutaneous manifestation of inflammatory intestinal disease. International Journal of Dermatology. 2013;**52**(12):1596-1598

Chapter 2

Behçet's Disease: An Enigmatic Malady with Plethoric Expressions

Shamaz Mohamed and Abhilash R. Krishnan

Abstract

Behçet's disease (BD) is a chronic, inflammatory, repetitive, debilitating systemic vasculitis with conglomerate system involvement of uncharted aetiology portrayed by the triad of oral ulcers, genital ulcers and cutaneous lesions. Behçet's disease has a universal distribution with a predominance among populace with higher prevalence of human leukocyte antigen (HLA) B5 and its split, HLA-B51, in the Mediterranean basin, the Middle East and Far East. This ailment is presently acknowledged to be a multisystem disorder with mucocutaneous, ocular, intestinal, articular, vascular, urogenital, musculoskeletal, cardiopulmonary and neurologic systems and hence bears significant organ sinistering morbidity and mortality. The diagnosis of Behçet's disease relies on scrupulous history, identification of its emblematic clinical countenance as per the diagnostic criteria construed by the International Study Group (ISG) and examination of all pertinent systems and excluding other systemic rheumatic diseases. However, there is a lag in diagnosis because of its plethoric presentations and a dearth of specific biomarkers. The multiple organ and tissue involvement of Behçet's disease necessitates an interdisciplinary approach from various health specialities since a general and an organ-specific approach is mandatory. Prime concern is to control the active periods of the disease which is achieved by different anti-inflammatory drugs, steroids or immunomodulators.

Keywords: Behçet's disease, triple symptom complex, Adamantiades-Behçet's disease, oral ulcers, aphthous stomatitis, vasculitis, silk road disease

1. Introduction

Behçet's disease (BD) is described as a severely debilitating chronic, recurrent, multisystem vascular inflammatory disorder characterised by the triad of oral and genital ulceration and ocular lesions. This exemplary presentation would have been probably first identified by Hippocrates [1, 2]. Even though Behçet's disease was first identified by the father of medicine in the fifth century BC, there were no literature representations for this entity till 1930, and then a Greek ophthalmologist Benediktos Adamantiades presented one of his case of relapsing eye lesions associated with genital ulceration and arthritis in a 20-year-old male; since then entity has been added with a synonym "Adamantiades-Behçet's disease" [3–6]. Further to its classic expression of orogenital ulceration and ocular lesions, the conditions seem to involve the musculoskeletal system, nervous system, gastrointestinal tract, vascular beds, urogenital tract and cardiopulmonary system, so Behçet's disease have a high morbidity and mortality particularly in males with early age onset [7, 8].

The self-limiting inflammation and the relapsing episodes of clinical manifestations are the hallmark of Behçet's disease [9]. Frequency and span of regression are uncertain and show no distinguishable pattern of onset.

Although Behçet's disease has a worldwide distribution, it is more rampant in Turkish population, where the prevalence is about 421 cases per 100,000 and 13 to 20 cases per 100,000 population in China, Korea, Japan and the Middle East [10, 11]. Behçet's disease is most commonly diagnosed in the second and third decades of life especially during the reproductive years and shows a female predilection among Europeans. Behçet's disease rarely occurs prior to puberty and after the fifth decade of life. Behçet's disease developing in early age has shown to have severe clinical manifestations and mortality. Familial occurrences have been reported in various literatures but are unusual, and the aetiology of Behçet's disease remains cryptic [12–18]. The widely accepted hypothesis is that of an inappropriate inflammatory response provoked by an infectious agent in a genetically liable host [19].

Diagnosis of Behçet's disease is based on the criteria developed by the International study group (ISG) in 1990 and International Criteria for Behçet's Disease (ICBD) [20]. The ICBD was developed with the intention of bettering the ISG criteria that did not consist of nervous system, vascular and gastrointestinal involvement that are severe but rather infrequent complications of Behçet's disease. A recent study conducted in the United Kingdom has compared the efficacy of ISG and ICBD diagnostic criteria among their patients with Behçet's disease and concluded that the sensitivity was higher for ICBD than ISG criteria, but the specificity of ICBD was much lower than the ISG criteria [20–22].

Management is aimed to alleviate symptoms, resolve inflammation, restrain tissue damage, dwindle frequency and severity and avoid lethal complications. A multitude of treatment modalities have been proposed for managing Behçet's disease ranging from anti-inflammatory to immunomodulators and biologic monoclonal antibodies. Detrimental ramifications are a main concern since it requires long-term medication [8].

2. Epidemiology

Behçet's disease is observed to have a worldwide distribution. However, it is seen commonly among the inhabitants of the historic Silk Road, which was supposed to be an old trading route that linked Japan and China in the Far East to the Mediterranean Sea, including countries such as Turkey and Iran. Therefore, Behçet's disease is also known by the synonym "Silk Road disease" [23]. Behçet's disease has a highest prevalence rate in Turkey, where the estimated prevalence is about 421 per 100,000 population followed by Iran, Israel and Japan [24]. It is rarely reported in African countries and the USA [23] as well as Australia, where the prevalence remains unknown but with an annual incidence of 0.6% (**Table 1**) [25].

Two studies conducted in Korea and Turkey in 2016 and 2017 reported the prevalence of Behçet's disease. A study conducted in Korea estimated the prevalence of Behçet's disease, and change in prevalence rate over time from the Korean healthcare big data that consists of medical institution claims data concerning diagnosis, prescription medicines and surgical treatment and represents the total population. The database was reviewed for patients diagnosed to have Behçet's disease during the year 2011 and 2015. The diagnosis was based on the Korean Standard Classification of Diseases (KCD). The estimated prevalence was about 35.0 per 100,000 population which was a little more than the previously reported prevalence of 30.2 per 100,000 in Korea. The change in prevalence rate was also estimated during the time period of 2011 and 2015 and concluded that there is a creeping

Prevalence per one lakh population	Country
Turkey	421
Iran	80
Saudi Arabia	20
Iraq	17
Israel	15.2
Japan	13.5
France	7.1
USA	5.2
Sweden	4.9
Germany	2.26
Portugal	1.53
UK	0.64

Table 1.
Worldwide prevalence of Behçet's disease [24].

escalation in the annual prevalence rate between 2011 and 2015. The prevalence rate was 32.8 per 100,000 in 2011, 34.0 per 100,000 in 2012, 34.6 per 100,000 in 2013, 35.5 per 100,000 in 2014 and 35.7 per 100,000 in 2015. The prevalence would have been more since patients with milder form of the disease have not come for treatment. Females had a higher prevalence, with a female-to-male ratio of 1:0.54 in 2011 and 1:0.56 in 2015 [26].

Another study conducted in Northern Turkey showed a prevalence of Behçet's disease in 600/100,000 population who have crossed their second decade of life and is considered as the highest prevalence reported in the literature so far [27]. Nonetheless this conclusion seems to be biased since there are methodological errors. Patients were randomly selected from the 52 urban and 33 rural general practices of a city and are invited for an examination and interview by three dermatologists. As per the authors, the invited sample would well represent the whole population since all individuals are recorded in general practices. Eye examination and pathergy test were performed in suspected individuals. Individuals compatible to ISG criteria were diagnosed as Behçet's disease. However, the total number of individuals who were invited for interview was not mentioned. Authors reported that 2325 of 2428 individuals interviewed were included in the study, of which 1290 were females and 1035 were males. Symptomatic individuals may have responded to the invitation, which might have led to a higher prevalence estimate. Authors have also reported increased prevalence of Behçet's disease in females (860/100,000) compared to males (140/100,000) ($p = 0.022$) which does not correlate with the previous studies conducted in Turkey, since they concluded no significant gender predilections [27].

A recent meta-analysis that included 45 prevalence studies suggested that even though there was clearly a wide variation across countries, the overall prevalence of Behçet's disease were 10.3/100,000. The estimated prevalence was 119.8/100,000 for Turkey, 31.8/100,000 for the Middle East, 4.5/100,000 for Asia and 3.3/100,000 for Europe [28]. A meta-regression analysis showed that classification criteria, study period or reference type had hardly any effect and study design was the deciding factor for Behçet's disease prevalence in these studies. The authors have also suggested that true geographic variations and different study methods are the possible factors responsible for the large variation in Behçet's disease prevalence across countries.

Two studies conducted in Korea reported on the clinical manifestations of Behçet's disease patients according to gender [29, 30]. The first study was carried out by a rheumatology department of a university hospital in Turkey, which assessed the prevalence between male and female with Behçet's disease in a retrospective chart review of 329 patients [29]. The study included patients who fulfilled the ISG criteria. Data on demographic features of the patients, family history, age of onset, manifestations of Behçet's, positive pathergy test and HLA-B51 were retrieved from patient charts. Among the 329 patients, 199 (60.4%) were males. A family history of Behçet's disease was reported by 9.7% of the patients and a family history of oral ulcers by 22.5%. Early onset was observed in patients with a positive family history; this phenomenon is termed as genetic anticipation which had already been seen in previous studies [31]. Female patients had an early onset compared to males (23.0 vs. 25.2 years, $p < 0.05$). Eye lesions were more common among males (42.2 vs. 29.2%, $p = 0.014$). Vascular involvement was also more common among in males (44.7 vs. 15.3%, $p < 0.001$), whereas joint involvement and headache were common among women (70.0 vs. 49.2%, $p < 0.001$ for joint involvement and 60.0 vs. 36.2%, $p < 0.001$ for headache). Frequency of genital ulcers, nodular lesions, papulo-pustular lesions and nervous system involvement was similar among males and females. Pathergy test was positive in 48.7% of the patients (52.4% among male and 43.4% among female, $p = 0.316$). HLA-B51 was positive in 44.1% of Behçet's disease patients, and the frequency was lower among men, but the difference was not that significant (38.8 vs. 50.6%, $p = 0.106$). The second study was conducted in Korea, which was a retrospective chart review of 193 patients, which analysed gender, age of onset of Behçet's disease and HLA-B51 [30]. The study showed that there is an increased prevalence in females (67%), whereas other parameters like the mean age at onset, the mean disease duration, positive pathergy test and positive HLA-B51 were similar in both males and females. Genital ulcers, peripheral joint involvement and inflammatory back pain were more common in females, while skin lesions were more frequent in males. In total, major organ involvement was present in 39% of the patients (uveitis, 27%; nervous system involvement, 7%; vascular involvement, 4% and gastrointestinal involvement, 11%), with similar frequency in both the genders. When clinical findings were compared based on onset of disease, patients with late onset (>40 years) had more nervous system involvement than those with an early onset (15.9 vs. 4.2%, $p = 0.007$).

Like the previous study, HLA-B51 positive patients had a history of early disease onset, but less nervous system (17.2 vs. 2.5%, $p = 0.02$) and gastrointestinal system (20.7 vs. 2.5%, $p = 0.01$) involvement than patients with negative HLA-B51 [32, 33].

A Japanese study conducted in 2015 analysed the change in disease phenotype over time among Behçet's disease patients treated in seven hospitals in a district in mid-Japan between 1991 and 2015. Patients fulfilled the 1987 revised diagnostic criteria of the Behçet's disease research committee; the Ministry of Health, Labour and Welfare of Japan was included in the study [34, 35]. This criterion classified the manifestations of Behçet's disease into major and minor symptoms. Major symptoms include recurrent aphthous oral ulcers, skin lesions, ocular inflammation and genital ulcers, and minor symptoms include arthritis, intestinal ulcers, epididymitis, vascular lesions and neuropsychiatric disease.

Those who have all four major symptoms during the clinical course are classified as complete, whereas those who have three major symptoms, two major and two minor symptoms, typical recurrent ocular inflammation and one or more major symptoms or typical recurrent ocular inflammation and two minor symptoms are classified as incomplete Behçet's disease. Patients were divided into three groups as group A, diagnosed before 2000; group B, diagnosed between 2000 and 2007; and group C, diagnosed after 2008. Authors observed a decrease in the number of patients with complete disease over time, suggesting a trend for milder disease in more recent years which could be due to usage of newer medicaments and awareness about the disease. The male-to-female ratio and the age of onset of disease were not changed over time, whereas the frequency of genital ulcers and HLA-B51 positivity decreased and gastrointestinal involvement frequency increased [34, 35].

Additionally, individuals migrated from countries with high prevalence of Behçet's disease to countries with less prevalence rate were shown to have less risk of developing disease [36, 37]. Prevalence of Behçet's disease among Turkish individuals in Germany is about 21/100,000, which, although higher than that of the German population, remains inferior to prevalence in Turkey [38].

Although Behçet's disease is rare in Africans, two series have been published recently based on studies conducted in Nigeria and Dakar from the year 2007 to 2011. Based on the observation by Italian authors, the prevalence of Behçet's disease was found to be higher among immigrants when they analysed its prevalence among patients of Italian and non-Italian origin living in these areas.

A study conducted in the Netherlands estimated the prevalence of Behçet's disease in patients with diverse ethnic origins residing in the Rotterdam area showed a prevalence of 1/100,000 population among Dutch Caucasians, 39/100,000 among Moroccans and 71/100,000 among Turks, suggesting that the prevalence among Moroccans is the same as in their countries of origin [39, 40].

3. Genetics

Peculiar geographical distribution, familial aggregation, polymorphisms in genes that control immune responses and correlation with HLA-B51 class I antigen are the four factors that are considered to contribute to Behçet's disease susceptibility. Ohno in 1973 described the association of BD with HLA-B5 [39]. They demonstrated that HLA-B5 includes HLA-B51 and HLA-B52 as it has a heterogeneous composition. In major histocompatibility locus, HLA-B51 and HLA-B5701 were associated with the pathogenesis of the disease, mainly among populace alongside of ancient Silk Road. Although associations with HLA-A and HLA-C have been described, they are non-specific and require confirmation. Other MHC genes such as TNF and MHC class I genes (MICA) are under study; the exact mechanism has not been fully understood. The association with HLA-B51 appears to be important in neutrophil activation. However, the presence of HLA-B51 alone is not ample to explain the manifestations of Behçet's disease. A case series of Iranian patients showed association with HLA-B35, HLA-B51, HLA-B52 and HLA-Bw4. Supplementary studies suggest associations with HLA-B15, HLA-B27, HLA-B57 and HLA-A26 [40].

Researches focused on single-nucleotide polymorphisms (SNPs) revealed that SNP which is in the HLA-B region between HLA-B and MICA genes is responsible for the relationship between HLA-B51 and Behçet's disease. The epistatic interactions with endoplasmic reticulum-associated aminopeptidase 1 (ERAP-1) has also been studied, and the authors suggested that the interaction of ERAP-1 and HLA-B has also been consistent, and these cytokines were apparently high in the peripheral blood mononuclear cells of patients with Behçet's disease compared to the control group. Another conclusion was the unbalanced suppressor of cytokine signalling expression in patients with Behçet's disease compared to controls [41].

A Chinese study stated that the polymorphisms of NOS3/rs1799983, a nitric oxide synthase gene, were found to be associated with the disease and the involvement of CD16 and CD11c in Behçet's disease susceptibility. Mutations in the familial Mediterranean fever (MEFV) gene were suggested by a meta-analysis of 8 studies which analysed 2538 patients and 2792 healthy controls. Researches also suggested the associations of Toll-like receptors 7 (TLR7) and other nucleic acid-sensing genes of innate immunity-like inflammatory pathways such as IFI16 (a dsDNA cytosolic sensor and mediator of the AIM2-dependent inflammatory pathway) found to influence Behçet's disease susceptibility [39]. Epigenetic studies with inverted repeat sequences (IRS) demonstrated that methylation level of IRS elements may influence the pathogenesis of the Behçet's disease. Researches were done on genes related to apoptosis, but the results were not conclusive [41].

4. Pathogenesis

A multitude of factors that indicate the interaction between environmental, innate and adaptive immunity in the development of the disease has been already discussed in the Genetics section. Various researches have studied about the role of bacterial and viral agents in the development of Behçet's disease, but the results were inconclusive. *Streptococcus sanguinis* and Herpesviridae were suspected as contributing extrinsic factors for the oral presentations in Behçet's disease; the immune response to these microorganisms and bacterial plaque ecology may be affected in Behçet's disease, leading to changes seen in the oral mucosa. However good prognosis was noticed in patients with good oral health status [41]. Recent studies in Behçet's disease patients have demonstrated peculiar dysbiosis of the gut microbial flora with a notable drop in the production of butyrate. Butyrate can initiate the differentiation of regulatory T cells (T-reg), and thus, its decrease would lead to the reduction of regulatory T-cell response and activation of immunopathological T-cell effector responses. Predisposition to insulin resistance and metabolic syndrome in patients and reduction of angiopoietin 1 especially in patients with vascular involvement has been observed in other studies [42]. In an attempt to find out specific Behçet's disease antigen, a Chinese research group demonstrated high IgG reactivity to an endothelial cell autoantigen [41].

Matzinger suggested the danger model, which occurs due to a continuous autoimmune cascade resulting from signals emitted by the affected cells of the host which will override the external stimulus. T cells and other antigen-presenting cells (APC) would command the process, which would be perpetuated on a favourable genetic terrain. Damage by a non-self-entity would trigger permanent aggression by activating an uncontrolled adaptive response. Because of their similarity to other pathogenic proteins, heat shock proteins (HSP60) could be involved. This adaptive reaction to external stimuli would persist in the permanent pathogenic presence via autoantigens that would activate dendritic T cells and B cells [40]. Thus, overexpression of proinflammatory cytokines especially Th1 and Th17 and probably association with genetic susceptibility may be the contributing factor for the increased inflammatory reaction in Behçet's disease. Stimulated lymphocytes would activate neutrophils and endothelial cells, and HSPs would probably trigger innate and adaptive immune responses. Hypersensitivity to *Streptococcus sanguinis* is observed through the innate immune system. Microbial flora along with stress proteins in oral and periodontal tissues could cross-react with host tissues and stimulate the proliferation of autoreactive T-cell clones. HSPs would transfer antigenic peptides to APCs that could be identified by TLRs, triggering an endogenous signal of danger that would lead to the activation of innate and adaptive immune systems. They could also, directly or indirectly, cause increased expression of vascular endothelial growth factor by T cells, causing both endothelial cell damage and vasculitis.

Many studies have demonstrated the presence of IFN-gamma and IL-12 in peripheral blood of Behçet's disease patients suggesting involvement of TH1 cells. Elevated IL-1, IL-6, IL-18, TNF-alpha and chemokines would reflect the activation of innate and adaptive immune systems. Neutrophils are hyperactivated with increased phagocytosis, chemotaxis, superoxide and lysosomal enzyme production. Lymphocytes have also shown abnormal functions such as clonal expansion of autoreactive T cells specific for heat shock protein 60 peptides. In addition, gamma-delta T cells are abundant in the blood and mucosal lesions of the affected individuals. Researchers have concluded that the interaction between T cells, neutrophils and antigen-presenting cells probably contributes to the pathogenesis of Behçet's disease [40].

5. Clinical presentations

Behçet's disease is a form of systemic vasculitis which affect almost all vascularized systems (**Table 2**) and is characterised by episodes of relapses and remissions [9, 43, 44].

The triad of oral aphthae, genital ulcers and ocular lesions specifies the disease pattern even though Behçet's disease has other multisystem involvement and several clinical manifestations.

Children exhibit more frequent perianal ulceration and more severe course of chorioretinitis and less frequent genital ulcers and vascular involvement [44, 45].

5.1 Eye manifestations

A meta-analysis of 18 articles which was performed by Horie et al. to assess the association between HLA-B51 and the ocular manifestations of Behçet's disease among various ethnic group studies from Middle and Far East suggested that there was a strong association between HLA-B51 expression and ocular involvement, whereas studies from North Africa and Europe showed no association [46].

Accorinti et al. investigated demographic and clinical trends of 385 Behçet's disease patients with uveitis seen over 44 years in a referral unit at Sapienza University in Rome, Italy. The cohort was divided into cohort 1, which included the patients seen from 1968 to 1992, and cohort 2 included the patients seen during 1993 and 2011. Compared to the cohort 1, the cohort 2 has more female patients, more patients with milder disease (more frequent isolated anterior uveitis, less frequent hypopyon) and more immunosuppressive use. Ocular complications such as optic atrophy, maculopathy and retinal neovascularisation and retinal detachment

Manifestation	Prevalence	Prognosis	Comments
Oral ulcers	47–83%	Favourable	Appear in all patients during the disease course
Genital ulcers	57–93%	Favourable	Lesion will leave a scar
Ocular lesions	30–70%	Poor	More frequent in males. Has high morbidity
Cutaneous lesions	38–99%	Favourable	Erythema nodosum more frequent in females
Joint involvement	45–60%	Favourable	Nondeforming and nonerosive
Cardiovascular involvement	7–49%	Poor	More frequent in males, high morbidity and mortality
Neurological involvement	5–10%	Poor	More frequent in males, high morbidity and mortality
Gastrointestinal involvement	3–26%	Poor	More frequent among Japanese

Table 2.
Manifestations of Behçet's disease.

were significantly more common in cohort 1. The visual acuity at final evaluation was better in the second cohort. When considered both the cohorts, more severe findings were observed in males. From the above findings, the authors concluded that timely and aggressive management reduces ocular complications and facilitates better prognosis [47].

Even though uveitis is the common ocular pathology in Behçet's disease, it is not a common cause of uveitis. The highest incidence of uveitis is reported by Mishima S from Japan [48], where it constitutes about 25%, but it is much rarer in other countries such as Brazil, where the incidence is 2% [49], and India, where the incidence is 1% reported by Sen DK from a study conducted in 94 Indian children [50]. The classical feature of Behçet's disease is recurrent, acute anterior uveitis associated with hypopyon. Other ocular manifestations seen in Behçet's disease include necrotizing vascular lesions involving the retina and the optic nerve. These manifestations may be unnoticed because of severity of the anterior segment reaction and commonly include macular oedema, retinal periphlebitis and periarteritis, thrombosis of the vessels and retinal or vitreous haemorrhages which are frequently observed in males with Behçet's disease [51, 52].

5.2 Oral manifestations

Recurrent oral ulcers are one of the earliest manifestations of Behçet's disease in around 47–86% of patients and are seen in almost all patients during their clinical course [53]. Other symptoms may at times take years to appear after the onset of disease. Oral ulcerative lesions usually manifest as a round- or oval-shaped ulcer with discrete erythematous border with a greyish-white pseudomembrane or a central yellowish fibrinous floor and grow rapidly from a flat ulcer to a deep sore [9]. They may occur as single ulcers or as numerous [9, 53]. Oral ulcers most commonly affect the gingival and buccal mucosa, tongue and lips yet may also appear in the soft and hard palates, pharynx and tonsils [9]. Minor ulcers which are less than 1 cm in diameter heal without scarring over a period of 1 to 2 weeks, whereas major ulcers which are more than 1 cm in diameter are more painful and heal within 2–6 weeks. Herpetiform ulcers occurring in recurrent crops of small ulcers that are 0.2–0.3 cm in diameter are painful and may coalesce to form large ulcers. Treatment is usually symptomatic, and prognosis of oral ulcerations is favourable [18, 53].

5.3 Cutaneous manifestations

The most commonly seen cutaneous manifestations are erythema nodosum and pseudofolliculitis, in which erythema nodosum is manifested as painful multiple subcutaneous nodules that vary in size and colour, whereas pseudofolliculitis (pustulosis) appears as a dome-shaped sterile pustule on a round reddish edematous base that looks like acne vulgaris [54]. Although these are commonly seen on the lower extremities, it can be seen throughout the body [55]. The pathergy reaction is included in the criteria for the diagnosis of Behçet's disease. Although more than 50% of patients from Turkey and Japan had a positive pathergy test, it is rarely observed in patients from Northern Europe, the USA and Australia [56, 57]. It used to be an important diagnostic criterion for Behçet's disease; however, the frequency of the pathergy phenomenon was reported to decrease during the recent years [58]. Subcutaneous thrombophlebitis is often confused with lesions of erythema nodosum; the former is manifested as tender erythematous nodules with a linear arrangement in most case. The lesions may relocate depending on the vascular segment involved [59].

5.4 Cardiac manifestations

Cardiac involvement is a rare finding in patients with Behçet's disease. Behçet's disease affects arteries, veins as well as the heart. Cardiovascular features have been reported to affect 7–49% of patients, more frequently in males. They occur 3–16 years after the onset of Behçet's disease. Cardiac involvement in Behçet's disease patients was first described by Mirone et al. in 1958 as a case of paroxysmal fibrillation and heart block. In 1963, Oshima et al. described a case of myocardial infarction complicated by incomplete right bundle-branch block [60]. Since then different types of cardiovascular lesions, including pericarditis, atrial thrombus, complex ventricular arrhythmia, myocardial infarction, heart block and sudden death, have been reported in association with Behçet's disease [61]. Dong Soo et al. in 1998 reported a case of superior vena cava syndrome caused by Behçet's disease in a 40-year-old man with recurrent oral aphthous ulcers and skin rashes on the anterior chest wall [62].

5.5 Neurological manifestations

Neurological involvement in Behçet's disease, the neuro-Behçet's disease, occurs very rarely and only in 5–10% of patients. It is frequently seen in males [63]. It usually occurs around 5 years after the onset of the disease and is associated with long-term morbidity and mortality [9]. Neuro-Behçet's disease can be parenchymal, nonparenchymal or mixed brain disease, in which the parenchymal brain disease affects the brainstem and/or basal ganglia and is correlated with a poor prognosis, whereas nonparenchymal also known as vasculo-Behçet's disease or angio-Behçet's disease is characterised by subsets of cerebral venous thromboses, dural venous sinus thrombosis, arterial vasculitis and aseptic meningitis and comprises the most devastating symptom category of Behçet's disease with high mortality [63, 64]. A mixed parenchymal and nonparenchymal disease has also been reported but is very rare. Infrequent clinical manifestations like epilepsy, stroke, brain tumour-like neuro-Behçet's disease, acute meningeal syndrome, movement disorders, optic neuropathy, spinal cord involvement and asymptomatic and subclinical neurological involvement have also been reported [65, 66]. Meningitis, neurological deficits including motor disturbances and brainstem symptoms and psychiatric symptoms including personality changes develop in patients with neuro-Behçet's disease are considered as a classic finding [18, 63]. These symptoms are associated with disease exacerbations and gradually cause disability and unfortunately are irreversible [18]. At late stages, dementia develops in approximately one-third of patients with neuro-Behçet's disease.

5.6 Gastrointestinal manifestations

Gastrointestinal involvement was observed in 3–26% of patients and varies among different populations [38, 39]. It is much more frequent in Japan than in the Middle East and the Mediterranean region [1–3]. Mucosal inflammation and ulceration can occur anywhere in the gastrointestinal tract but typically in the ileocecal region. Other rarely involved sites include the oesophagus, ascending colon and transverse colon [18, 19, 67]. Clinical symptoms include anorexia, vomiting, dyspepsia, diarrhoea, melena, abdominal pain and, less frequently, perforation requiring surgical intervention [68]. Due to the similarity in intestinal and extraintestinal symptoms, it is tough to differentiate Behçet's disease from inflammatory bowel disease; however, the presence of granulomata can be used to confirm inflammatory bowel disease [66].

5.7 Articular manifestations

Joint involvement is common in patients with Behçet's disease seen in almost half of patients. It presents as an initial manifestation seen long before the commencement of other features of BD [55]. Erosive, non-deforming oligoarthritis typically involving the knees, ankles and wrists is seen in most of the Behçet's disease patients. Rarely, it can present as sacroiliitis or erosive arthritis. Myopathy has also been reported by Arkin in 1980 [69–72].

5.8 Vascular manifestations

Vasculitis is one of the classic signs in Behçet's disease, and the typical finding is deep vein thrombosis. Thrombophlebitis occurs generally in the first year after onset of Behçet's disease, and relapses are frequent. Vasculitis can affect both the veins and arteries and capillaries although venous involvement is more common [55]. Venous thrombosis may occur at any site and can even involve large vessels like the inferior vena cava, the superior vena cava and the pulmonary artery. [55]. Arterial involvement is seen in 3–5% of cases [73]. Aneurysm formation is found to be the foremost manifestation, and the affected patients can be asymptomatic [74]. Vascular surgery is mandatory, but relapse is a frequent concern [55].

5.9 Pulmonary manifestations

Pulmonary manifestations are rare in patients with Behçet's disease. Haemoptysis is the only reported manifestation, but it can be massive and fatal [74].

6. Diagnostic criterion and activation markers in Behçet's disease

The diagnosis of Behçet's disease relies purely on its clinical manifestation since it lacks specific biological test, so diagnosis with clinical symptoms is challenging, especially due to non-concomitant symptoms. Hence different diagnostic criteria have been developed for the determination of Behçet's disease. In 1990, an ISG for Behçet's disease was formed by a group of researchers [21]. The International Study Group developed a set of classification criteria which is designed for research studies, which in many instances is used for diagnosing. The features were defined as the presence of specific symptoms as seen in **Table 3**. Oral ulceration along with any other two symptoms is said to be diagnostic [75]. The capability of the ISG criteria as a diagnostic tool has been questioned [56]. An international team which includes 27 countries was formed to evaluate and reassess the ISG criteria, and a new ICBD was developed that include the major criteria consisting of oral aphthosis, genital aphthosis and ocular lesions which were each given 2 points, whereas 1 point was assigned to the skin lesion, neurological manifestation, vascular manifestation and positive pathergy test (which is optional and not included in the primary criteria due to geographic variation and its declining sensitivity and increased specificity) [58, 75]. Higher sensitivity of the ICBD was reported as it aided in earlier diagnosis and hence earlier treatment and thereby better prognosis [75]. However, the delay between the onsets of major manifestations may be decades needs to be considered [76]. Inflammatory markers such erythrocyte sedimentation rate (ESR) and C-reactive protein have no longer been recognised as accurate or specific for the disease activity (**Table 4**).

Investigations for Behçet's disease include routine total blood count; renal, liver and bone profile; inflammatory markers, including C-reactive protein and erythrocyte sedimentation rate; urine analysis; chest X-ray; coeliac screen; stool sample; autoimmune

Recurrent oral ulcerations	Minor aphthous, major aphthous or herpetiform ulceration observed by physician or patient, which recurred at least three times in one 12-month period
Plus any two of the following	
Recurrent genital ulceration	Aphthous ulceration or scarring observed by physician or patient
Eye lesion	Anterior uveitis, posterior uveitis or cells in vitreous on slit lamp examination or retinal vasculitis observed by ophthalmologist
Skin lesions	Erythema nodosum observed by physician or patient, pseudofolliculitis or papulopustular lesions or acneiform nodules observed by physician in post adolescent patients not on corticosteroid treatment
Positive pathergy test	Read by a physician at 24–48 hours

Table 3.
The international study group criteria for Behçet's disease [21].

Symptoms	Points
Oral aphthosis	2
Genital aphthosis	2
Ocular lesion	2
Skin lesion	1
Neurological manifestation	1
Vascular manifestation	1
Positive pathergy test	1[b]

Table 4.
International criteria for Behçet's disease [75].

screen; coagulation profile and antiphospholipid antibodies; mouth and genital ulcer swab and culture; and occasionally eye swab. Other investigations that may be required include oral biopsy and direct immunofluorescence to exclude orofacial granulomatosis and bullous dermatosis. Vulval biopsy is indicated to exclude lichen sclerosis).

Doppler studies, CT or MRI brain and spinal cord, magnetic resonance venography, computerised tomographic venography, magnetic resonance angiography, computerised tomography angiography to evaluate neurologic and vascular disease; CSF studies, electro encephalogram, electromyography, nerve conduction study, 18 F fluoro2-deoxyglucose positron emission tomography, with CT/MRI localisation (for early inflammation in large vessel vasculitis). Musculoskeletal BD—synovial fluid analysis, X-ray, ultrasound or MRI to evaluate joints. Skin biopsy and immunofluorescence for cutaneous involvement. Cardiac BD—electrocardiogram, echocardiogram in case of cardio vascular involvement chest CT to assess mediastinal diseases, fibrosing mediastinitis, aneurysms, pleural effusions, complications of venous thrombosis and collaterals. Stool sample for faecal calprotectin, endoscopy and biopsy if there is Gastrointestinal involvement. Ocular BD—optical coherence tomography, visual evoked potentials, fluorescein angiogram, Schirmer's test, intraocular fluid culture to exclude infections in Behçets patients with ocular involvement. Cystoscopy and kidney, urinary bladder CT for urological disease [7].

7. Management

The multisystem involvement in Behçet's systems alarms the requirement of a teamwork from different medical specialties such as oral medicine, ophthalmology,

Manifestations	Treatments
Mild mucocutaneous lesions	Topical steroids
Moderate to severe mucocutaneous lesions	Initial: systemic steroid, colchicine
	Refractory case: azathioprine, interferonα
Ocular lesions	Initial: systemic steroid + azathioprine
	Refractory case: first cyclosporine A + steroid + azathioprine Second interferon α+/− systemic steroid
Arthritis	(First) colchicine nonsteroidal anti-inflammatory drug, (second) azathioprine, interferon α
Vascular: deep venous thrombosis	Azathioprine, cyclosporine A, cyclophosphamide (larger vessels)
Vascular: arterial aneurysm	Cyclophosphamide + systemic steroid
Neurological	Cyclophosphamide (drug of choice)
Gastrointestinal	Systemic steroid, sulfasalazine, azathioprine

Table 5.
Suggested management options of Behçet's disease [78, 79].

Disease-modifying drugs (DMDs)	Dosage
Oral DMDs	
Azathioprine	2–3 mg/kg/day
Mycophenolate mofetil	2–3 g/day
Methotrexate	20–25 mg/week
Tacrolimus	4–8 mg/day
Ciclosporin	2–5 mg/kg/day
Sulfasalazine	2–3 g/day
Dapsone	2–3 mg/kg/day
Thalidomide (exceptional use)	50–300 mg/day
Colchicine	0.5–2 mg/day
Prednisolone	Variable dose (depending on indication and stage of treatment)
Parenteral DMDs	
Cyclophosphamide	15 mg/kg (vasculitis regimens)
Anti-TNF α inhibitors	
Infliximab	5 mg/kg at 0, 2 and 6 weeks then once every 8 weeks
Adalimumab	40 mg every 2 weeks
Etanercept	50 mg/week
Certolizumab	400 mg at 0, 2 and 4 weeks then once every 4 week
Rituximab	1 g at 0 and 2 weeks
Interferon α	Various regimens for Roferon A and pegylated interferon α 2b
Alemtuzumab	3 mg (day 1), 10 mg (day 3), 30 mg (day 5), 30 mg (day 8), 30 mg (day 10) and 30 mg (day 12)

Table 6.
Disease-modifying drugs used in Behçet's disease [7].

DOI: http://dx.doi.org/10.5772/intechopen.86863

dermatology, rheumatology, neurology, cardiology and gastroenterology for its management. The main objective of management of Behçet's disease is to induce and maintain remission and improve the patient's quality of life, preventing irreversible damage and exacerbation of mucocutaneous and articular disease [77, 78]. Since Behçet's disease has plethoric expressions, treatment plan may vary depending on severity, organ affected, age of disease onset, disease duration and frequency of recurrences [59].

The European League Against Rheumatism (EULAR) formed a committee in 2008 to develop an evidence-based recommendation for the treatment modalities of Behçet's disease [78]. Suggestions regarding ocular and mucocutaneous diseases and arthritis are primarily evidence-based, but recommendations on neurological, vascular and gastrointestinal involvement relied on observational studies, retrospective analyses and expert opinion [78].

Treatment of Behçet's disease is mainly based on the suppression of the inflammatory attack using immunomodulatory agents such as corticosteroids, azathioprine or interferon α [78]. The primary line of management of mucocutaneous lesions in Behçet's disease is colchicine (1 mg/day). NSAID is usually sufficient for joint manifestations [54]. Clinicians should keep in mind the neurotoxicity of cyclosporine A while prescribing it to any patient with neurologic problems for treating vascular involvement and refractory eye disease [54]. Biologic agents are the only option if the disease seems to be resistant to treatments [78]. Suggested management options are summarised in **Tables 5** and **6**.

8. Conclusion

Behçet's disease is a chronic, relapsing vasculitis with multisystem involvement with considerable morbidity and mortality. There exists a delay in the diagnosis of Behçet's disease since it lacks a specific diagnostic test and biomarkers. Another area to be focussed on is to develop a more effective disease activity score. Researches are on the go to explore more about the disease's pathophysiology which may aid in early diagnosing and effective treatment planning.

Acknowledgements

We thank Prof Dr. Sobha Kuriakose, Dr. Sarika S. Kamal, Dr. Sumal V. Raj, Dr. Nithin V. S and Dr. Deena C. Thomas, Dr. Alaka Subodh and Adithi S. A for critically analysing this manuscript.

Author details

Shamaz Mohamed* and Abhilash R. Krishnan
Sri Sankara Dental College, India

*Address all correspondence to: shamazmohamed@gmail.com

References

[1] Feigenbaum A. Description of Behçets syndrome in the hippocratic third book of endemic diseases. The British Journal of Ophthalmology. 1956;**40**:355-357

[2] Rohatgi J, Singal A. Ocular manifestations of Behçets disease in Indian patients. Indian Journal of Ophthalmology. 2003;**51**:309-313

[3] Martineau M, Haskard DO, Nelson-Piercy C. Behçet's syndrome in pregnancy. Obstetric Medicine. 2010;**3**:2-7

[4] Eguia A, Villarroel M, Martínez-Conde R, Echebarría MÁ, Aguirre JM. Adamantiades-Behçet disease: An enigmatic process with oral manifestations. Medicina Oral Patología Oral y Cirugía Bucal. 2006;**11**:E6-E11

[5] Leonardo NM, McNeil J. Behçet's disease. Is there geographical variation? A review far from the silk road. International Journal of Rheumatology. 2015;**2015**:1-7

[6] Zouboulis CC, Keitel W. A historical review of early descriptions of Adamantiades-Behçet's disease. The Journal of Investigative Dermatology. 2002;**119**:201-205

[7] Nair JR, Moots RJ. Behçet's disease. Clinical Medicine. 2017;**17**(1):71-77

[8] Zeidan MJ, Saadoun D, Garrido M, Klatzmann D, Six A, Cacoub P. Behçet's disease physiopathology: A contemporary review. Autoimmunity Highlights. 2016;**7**(4):1-12

[9] Mendes D, Correia M, Barbedo M, Vaio T, Mota M, Gonçalves O, et al. Behçet's disease—A contemporary review. Journal of Autoimmunity. 2009;**32**(3-4):178-188

[10] Tsuyoshi S, Mitsuhiro T. Behçet's disease current concepts. The New England Journal of Medicine. 1999;**341**:1284-1291

[11] Escudier M, Bagan J, Scully C. Behçet's disease (Adamantiades syndrome). Oral Diseases. 2006;**12**:78-84

[12] Fenech FF, Soler NG. Behçet's syndrome with neurological manifestations in two sisters. British Medical Journal. 1968;**2**:472-473

[13] Goolamali SK, Comaish JS, Hassanyeh F, Stephens A. Familial Behçet's syndrome. The British Journal of Dermatology. 1976;**95**:637-642

[14] Abdel-Aziz AM, Fairburn EA. Familial Behçet's syndrome. Cutis. 1978;**21**:649-652

[15] Berman L, Trappler B, Jenkins T. Behçet's syndrome: A family study and elucidation of a genetic role. Annals of the Rheumatic Diseases. 1979;**38**:118-121

[16] Kobayashi T, Sudo Y, Okamura S. Monozygotic twins concordant for intestinal Behçet's disease. Journal of Gastroenterology. 2005;**40**:4

[17] Saadoun D, Wechsler B, Desseaux K, Le Thi Huong D, Amoura Z, Resche-Rigon M, et al. Mortality in Behçet's disease. Arthritis and Rheumatism. 2010;**62**(9):2806-2812

[18] Sakane T, Takeno M, Suzuki N. Behçet's disease. The New England Journal of Medicine. 1999;**341**(17):1284-1291

[19] Marshall SE. Behçet's disease. Best Practice & Research Clinical Rheumatology. 2004;**18**:291-311

[20] Blake T, Pickup L, Carruthers D. Birmingham Behçet's service: Classification of disease and application of the 2014 international criteria for Behçet's disease (ICBD) to a UK cohort.

BMC Musculoskeletal Disorders. 2017;**18**:101-113

[21] InternatIonal Study group for Behçet's disease. Criteria for the diagnosis of Behçet's disease. Lancet. 1990;**335**:1078-1080

[22] Davatchi F, Assaad Khalil S, Calamia KT. The international criteria for Behçet's disease (ICBD): A collaborative study of 27 countries on the sensitivity and specificity of the new criteria. Journal of the European Academy of Dermatology and Venereology. 2014;**28**:338-347

[23] Keinoand H, Okada A. Behçet's disease: Global epidemiology of an old silk road disease. The British Journal of Ophthalmology. 2007;**91**:1573-1574

[24] Mohammad A, Mandl T, Sturfelt G, Segelmark M. Incidence, prevalence and clinical characteristics of Behçet's disease in southern Sweden. Rheumatology. 2013;**52**(2):304-310

[25] Wakefieldand D, Mc Cluskey P. Behçet's syndrome: Ocular features in an Australian population. Australian and New Zealand Journal of Ophthalmology. 1990;**18**(2):129-135

[26] Kim JN, Kwak SG, Choe JY, Kim SK. The prevalence of Behçet's disease in Korea: Data from Health Insurance Review and Assessment Service from 2011 to 2015. Clinical and Experimental Rheumatology. 2017;**35**(108):38-42

[27] Baş Y, Seçkin HY, Kalkan G. Investigation of Behçet's disease and recurrent aphthous stomatitis frequency: The highest prevalence in Turkey. Balkan Medical Journal. 2016;**33**:390-395

[28] Maldini C, Druce K, Basu N, Lavalley MP, Mahr A. Exploring the variability in Behçet's disease prevalence: A meta-analytical approach. Rheumatology. 2018;**57**(1):185-195

[29] Dü C, Kaşifoğlu T, Korkmaz C. Do clinical findings of Behçet's disease vary by gender? A single-centre experience from 329 patients. European Journal of Rheumatology. 2016;**3**:157-160

[30] Ryu HJ, Seo MR, Choi HJ, Baek HJ. Clinical phenotypes of Korean patients with Behçet disease according to gender, age at onset, and HLA-B51. The Korean Journal of Internal Medicine. 2018;**33**(5):1025-1031

[31] Fresko I, Soy M, Hamuryudan V. Genetic anticipation in Behçet's syndrome. Annals of the Rheumatic Diseases. 1998;**57**:45-48

[32] Yoshida A, Kawashima H, Motoyama Y. Comparison of patients with Behçet's disease in the 1980s and 1990s. Ophthalmology. 2004;**111**:810-815

[33] Cingu AK, Onal S, Urgancioglu M, Tugal-Tutkun I. Comparison of presenting features and three-year disease course in Turkish patients with Behçet uveitis who presented in the early 1990s and the early 2000s. Ocular Immunology and Inflammation. 2012;**20**:423-428

[34] Kirino Y, Ideguchi H, Takeno M. Continuous evolution of clinical phenotype in 578 Japanese patients with Behçet's disease: A retrospective observational study. Arthritis Research & Therapy. 2016;**18**:217

[35] Mizushima Y, Inaba G, Mimura Y. Guide for the diagnosis of Behçet's disease. In: Report of Behçet's Disease Research, Japan. 1987. pp. 8-17

[36] Verity DH, Marr JE, Ohno S, Wallace GR, Stanford MR. Behçet's disease, the silk road and HLA-B51: Historical and geographical perspectives. Tissue Antigens. 1999;**54**(3):213-220

[37] Yazici H, Akokan G, Yalçin B, Müftüoğlu A. The high prevalence of

HLA-B5 in Behçet's disease. Clinical and Experimental Immunology. 1977;**30**(2):259-261

[38] Savey L, Resche-Rigon M, Wechsler B, Comarmond C, Piette JC, Cacoub P, et al. Ethnicity and association with disease manifestations and mortality in Behçet's disease. Orphanet Journal of Rare Diseases. 2014;**27**(9):42

[39] Scherrer MAR, Rocha VB, Garcia LC. Behçet's disease: Review with emphasis on dermatological aspects. Anais Brasileiros de Dermatologia. 2017;**92**(4):452-464

[40] Zeidan MJ, Saadoun D, Garrido M, Klatzmann D, Six A, Cacoub P. Behçet's disease physiopathology: A contemporary review. Autoimmunity Highlights. 2016;**7**:4

[41] Hatemi G, Seyahi E, Fresko I, Talarico R, Hamuryudan V. One year in review 2016: Behçet's syndrome. Clinical and Experimental Rheumatology. 2016;**34**:10-22

[42] Hatemi G, Seyahi E, Fresko I, Talarico R, Hamuryudan V. Behçet's syndrome: A critical digest of the 2014-2015 literature. Clinical and Experimental Rheumatology. 2015;**33**:S3-S14

[43] Sfikakis PP, Markomichelakis N, Alpsoy E, Assaad-Khalil S, Bodaghi B, Gul A. Anti-TNF therapy in the management of Behçet's disease-review and basis for recommendations. Rheumatology. 2007;**46**(5):736-741

[44] Sfikakis PP. Behçet's disease: A new target for anti-tumor necrosis factor treatment. Annals of the Rheumatic Diseases. 2002;**61**(2):51-53

[45] Gul A, Inanc M, Ocal L, Aral O, Konice M. Familial aggregation of Behçet's disease in Turkey. Annals of the Rheumatic Diseases. 2000;**59**(8):622-625

[46] Horie Y, Meguro A, Ohta T. HLAB51 carriers are susceptible to ocular symptoms of Behçet disease and the association between the two becomes stronger towards the east along the silk road: A literature survey. Ocular Immunology and Inflammation. 2017;**25**:37-40

[47] Accorinti M, Pesci FR, Pirraglia MP, Abicca I, Pivetti-Pezzi P. Ocular Behçet's disease: Changing patterns over time, complications and long-term visual prognosis. Ocular Immunology and Inflammation. 2017;**25**:29-36

[48] Mishima S, Masuda K, Izawa Y, Mochizuki M, Namba K. Behçets disease in Japan: Ophthalmological aspects. Transactions of the American Ophthalmological Society. 1979;**77**:225-279

[49] Barra C, Belfort R, Abreu MT, Kim MK, Martins MC, Petrilli AMN. Behçet's disease in Brazil: A review of 49 cases with emphasis on ophthalmic manifestation. Japanese Journal of Ophthalmology. 1991;**35**:339-346

[50] Sen DK. Endogenous uveitis in Indian children: Analysis of 94 cases. Journal of Pediatric Ophthalmology. 1976;**14**:25-32

[51] Ames PR, Steuer A, Pap A, Denman AM. Thrombosis in Behçets disease: A retrospective survey from a single UK centre. Rheumatology. 2001;**40**:652-655

[52] Ermakova NA, Alekberova ZS. Retinal vasculitis in Behçets disease. Vestnik Oftalmologii. 2001;**117**:44-46

[53] Alpsoy E, Donmez L, Bacanli A, Apaydin C, Butun B. Review of the chronology of clinical manifestations in 60 patients with Behçet's disease. Dermatology. 2003;**4**:354-356

[54] Davatchi F, Shahram F, Chams Davatchi C. Behçet's disease: From

east to west. Clinical Rheumatology. 2010;**29**(8):823-833

[55] Saadounand D, Wechsler B. Behçet's disease. Orphanet Journal of Rare Diseases. 2012;**7**(1):20

[56] Varol A, Seifert O, Anderson CD. The skin pathergy test: Innately useful? Archives of Dermatological Research. 2010;**302**(3):155-168

[57] Altac M, Tuzun Y, Yurdakul S, Binyildiz P, Yazici H. The validity of the pathergy test (non-specific skin hyper reactivity) in Behçet's disease: A double-blind study by independent observers. Acta Dermato-Venereologica. 1982;**62**(2):158-159

[58] Davatchi F, Chams-Davatchi C, Ghodsi Z. Diagnostic value of pathergy test in Behçet's disease according to the change of incidence over the time. Clinical Rheumatology. 2011;**30**(9):1151-1155

[59] Alpsoy E. Behçet's disease: A comprehensive review with a focus on epidemiology, etiology and clinical features, and management of mucocutaneous lesions. The Journal of Dermatology. 2016;**43**:620-632

[60] Mirone L, Altomonte L, Ferlisi EM, Zoli A, Magaró M. Behçet's disease and cardiac arrhythmia. Clinical Rheumatology. 1997;**16**(1):99-100

[61] Kaya EB, Yorgun H, Akdoganetal A. Heart-rate recovery index is impaired in Behçet's disease. Texas Heart Institute Journal. 2009;**36**(4): 282-286

[62] Han DS. A case of Behçet's syndrome with superior vena cava syndrome. The Korean Journal of Internal Medicine. 1998;**13**(1):72-75

[63] Arai Y, Kohno S, Takahashi Y, Miyajima Y, Tsutusi Y. Autopsy case of neuro-Behçet's disease with multifocal neutrophilic perivascular inflammation. Neuropathology. 2006;**26**(6):579-585

[64] Hadfield MG, Aydin A, Lippman HR, Sanders KM. Neuro-Behçet's disease. Clinical Neuropathology. 1997;**16**(2):55-60

[65] Kidd D. Neurological complications of Behçet's syndrome. Current Neurology and Neuroscience Reports. 2012;**12**(6):675-679

[66] Saadoun D, Wechsler B, Resche-Rigon M, Trad S, Le Thi Huong D, Sbai A. Cerebral venous thrombosis in Behçet's disease. Arthritis and Rheumatism. 2009;**61**(4):518-526

[67] Lee KS, Kim SJ, Lee BC, Yoon DS, Lee WJ, Chi HS. Surgical treatment of intestinal Behçet's disease. Yonsei Medical Journal. 1997;**38**(6):455-460

[68] Beales IL. Gastrointestinal involvement in Behçet's syndrome. The American Journal of Gastroenterology. 1998;**93**(12):26-33

[69] Düzgün N, Ateş A. Erosive arthritis in a patient with Behçet's disease. Rheumatology International. 2003;**23**(5):265-267

[70] Benamour S, Zeroual B, Alaoui F-Z. Joint manifestations in Behçet's disease: A review of 340 cases. Revue du Rhumatisme. 1998;**65**(5):299-307

[71] El Maghraoui A, Tabache F, Bezzaetal A. A controlled study of sacroiliitis in Behçet's disease. Clinical Rheumatology. 2001;**20**(3):189-191

[72] Arkin C, Rothschild B, Fluorendo N, Popoff N. Myopathy in Behçet syndrome. Arthritis & Rheumatology. 1980;**23**:600-604

[73] Saadoun D, Asli B, Wechsler B. Long-term outcome of arterial lesions in Behçet disease: A series of 101 patients. Medicine. 2012;**91**(1):18-24

[74] Hamuryudan V, Er T, Seyahi E. Pulmonary artery aneurysms in Behçet syndrome. The American Journal of Medicine. 2004;**117**(11):867-870

[75] International Team for the Revision of the International Criteria for Behçet's Disease (ITR-ICBD). The International Criteria for Behçet's Disease (ICBD): A collaborative study of 27 countries on the sensitivity and specificity of the new criteria. Journal of the European Academy of Dermatology and Venereology. 2014;**28**(3):338-347

[76] Kitaichi N, Miyazaki A, Iwata D, Ohno S, Stanford MR, Chams H. Ocular features of Behçet's disease: An international collaborative study. The British Journal of Ophthalmology. 2007;**91**(12):1579-1582

[77] Saleh Z, Arayssi T. Update on the therapy of Behçet disease. Therapeutic Advances in Chronic Disease. 2014;**5**:112-134

[78] Hatemi G, Silman A, Bang D, Bodaghi B, Chamberlain AM, Gul A. ELAR recommendations for the management of Behçet disease. Annals of the Rheumatic Diseases. 2008;**67**:1656-1662

[79] Barry RJ, Markandey B, Malhotra R. Evidence-based practice in Behçet's disease: Identifying areas of unmet need for 2014. Orphanet Journal of Rare Diseases. 2014;**9**(1):16

Section 2

Pathogenesis of Behçet's Disease

Chapter 3

Genetics of Behçet's Disease

Xiaodong Zhou and Yan Deng

Abstract

Behçet's disease (BD) is a chronic refractory multi-system autoimmune disorder with a strong genetic component. Like many other human complex diseases, multiple genes with polymorphisms have been associated with BD. These genes encode proteins involved mainly in immune regulation and inflammation and some in transcriptional activation and post-translational modification. Understanding the genetic association of these genes with BD may provide insight into the pathogenesis and for development of new, targeted therapies for this human complex disease.

Keywords: Behçet's disease, genetic, HLA region, interleukin family, inflammation and autoimmunity, transcriptional activation

1. Introduction

Behçet's disease (BD) is a chronic inflammatory disorder with unclear etiology. It can affect a variety of organs characterized by refractory ulcers in genitals and mouth, uveitis, skin lesions, and manifestations in joints, gastrointestinal tract, kidneys, lungs, and cardiovascular and central nervous systems [1]. BD has distinctive geographical distribution, and it is found primarily in populations along the ancient Silk Route from the Mediterranean region transiting through Central Asia to East Asia [2]. The reported prevalence of BD varies between Western (0.12–7.5 per 100,000) [3] and Eastern countries (6.3–14 per 100,000) [4]. Turkey has the highest incidence of BD in general population (80–420 per 100,000) [5–7]. A family history of BD significantly increases the risk at a rate of 31.2% [8], which indicates a strong genetic contribution to the disease by comparing to general population. Men are more commonly affected in Middle Eastern countries, but that appears opposite in USA, Brazil, Israel, and Korea [9]. The first reported genetic association of BD was found in the human leukocyte antigen (HLA) region, or the major histocompatibility complex (MHC) on chromosome 6 [10]. HLA-B51 confers the strongest genetic risk to BD [11]. Multiple other genetic factors outside the HLA region have also been identified. The following are the categorized genes associated with BD reported from 1973 to January 2019.

2. HLA and HLA-related genes

2.1 HLA

HLA genes are among the most polymorphic genes in the human genome, and they are associated with almost all autoimmune diseases. HLA-B51 is the strongest risk allele for BD, which has been replicated in almost all studied populations [12–22]. The population attributable risk (PAR) of HLA-B5/B51 was estimated as 52.2% for BD

IntechOpen

patients in Southern Europe, 49.9% in Middle East/North Africa, 44.4% in East Asia, and 31.7% in Northern Europe [23]. Other HLA alleles including BD-risk HLA-A02, -A24, -A26, -A31, -B27, -B57, and BD-protective HLA-A03, -B15, -B35, -B49, -B58 were reported in different populations [22, 24–29].

Certain HLA alleles were also associated with clinical outcomes of BD. BD patients carrying HLA-A26:01 have a poor visual prognosis in Japan [30] and a high incidence of posterior uveitis in Korea [31]. Some HLA alleles were associated with lesions of specific organs in the Korean and Japanese patients, such as HLA-A26:01 with uveitis, HLA-A02:07 with skin lesions and arthritis, and -A30:04 with vascular lesions, genital ulcers, and a positive pathergy test [32]. These findings suggest that specific HLA alleles are likely used as genetic markers for subclassification and/or prognostic evaluation of BD patients.

2.2 CIITA

The class II major histocompatibility complex transactivator (CIITA) is a transcriptional activator that acts as a master regulator of the HLA class II genes and some other immune-mediating genes [33, 34]. A single nucleotide polymorphism (SNP) of the CIITA gene rs12932187 with G allele and GG genotype appeared to be a risk factor to Chinese BD, and the GG carriers were correlated with a higher expression of the CIITA gene, and with a lower level of IL-10 protein from the peripheral blood mononuclear cells (PBMC) in response to lipopolysaccharide (LPS) [35].

2.3 ERAP1

Endoplasmic reticulum aminopeptidase 1 (ERAP1) is an essential enzyme to trim peptides in the ER for optimized binding by MHC class I molecules. The association between ERAP1 and BD was first reported in a Turkish population and was replicated in a Chinese cohort, in which the SNPs rs10050860 and rs17482078 of the ERAP1 gene encoding variants of amino acids Asp575Asn and Arg725Gln, respectively, conferred risk to BD [36, 37]. Further analysis of the association indicated that the ERAP1 variant Arg725Gln may interact with the HLA-B51 protein to confer susceptibility to BD [36, 38]. Moreover, the expression of ERAP1 was found to be significantly lower in active BD patients [37], and the patients carrying AA and CC genotype of the ERAP1 SNP rs1065407 and rs10050860, respectively, showed a higher expression level of the ERAP1 gene than the patients carrying AC or CC and CT or TT genotypes of the SNPs, respectively, in response to LPS [37, 38].

2.4 MICA

The major histocompatibility complex class I chain-related gene A (MICA), located on the centromeric side of the HLA-B gene on chromosome 6, is highly polymorphic [39]. It functions in immune activation under cellular stress conditions, such as infections, tissue injury, pro-inflammatory signals, and malignant transformation [40]. There have been more than 100 MICA alleles identified according to its overall sequence variations. In addition, the codon 295 of the MICA gene has a tri-nucleotide microsatellite polymorphism (GCT)n that is designated as An (A4, A5, A6, A9) allele, and a five repetition of GCT may coexist with a guanosine insertion that is designated as A5.1 [41].

MICA*009 and *019 alleles were associated with BD in a Spanish population [42], and MICA-A6 allele with Japanese and Korean BD patients [43–45]. The latter appeared to be independent from the potential linkage disequilibrium (LD) effect of HLA-B51 according to the Korean study [45].

On the other hand, MICA-A5.1 demonstrated a negative correlation with ocular lesions and iridocyclitis in BD patients [45, 46]. MICA-A9 was associated with BD patients who had less severe complications including uveitis, thrombosis, and neurological and intestinal involvement [47].

3. Interleukin (IL) family genes

3.1 IL-10

IL-10 is a cytokine with anti-inflammatory properties, which plays critical roles in modulating immune response and preventing inflammatory and autoimmune pathologies [48, 49]. The SNP rs1800871 of the IL10 promoter region was first found in an association with BD in the UK and Middle Eastern (ME) cohorts [50]. The genome-wide association studies (GWAS) revealed multiple BD-associated SNPs (rs1518111, rs1554286, rs1800871, and rs1800872) of the IL-10 in Chinese, Turkey, Japanese, and Korean cohorts [51–53].

3.2 IL-12A, IL-23R, and IL-12RB2

IL-12A is a gene which encodes for IL-35 that is a subunit of the heterodimeric cytokines IL-12 (encoded by IL-12B) and IL-35. IL-35 binds to a heterodimeric IL-12 receptor (IL-12R) that consists of IL-12Rβ1 (encoded by IL-12RB1) and IL-12Rβ2 (encoded by IL-12RB2) [54], and it impacts on activation of NK cells and polarization of the Th1 pathway through differentiation from naïve CD4+ T cells [55, 56]. The association of the IL-12A variants rs1780546 and rs17810458 with BD was found in the Turkish and European cohorts [36, 57].

IL-23 is a member of the IL-12 cytokine family. It plays crucial roles in the development process of the Th17 cells [58]. The receptor for IL-23 is composed of two subunits encoded by the IL-23R and the IL-12RB1 genes [59], and it plays a key role in neutrophil inflammation and in autoimmune diseases [60].

A significant association (reaching a GWAS p value) of the IL-23R gene with BD was found at the SNP rs11209026 (Gly149Arg) in Japanese, and at the SNP rs76418789 (Arg381Gln) in Turkish cohort [61]. The association between BD and the IL-23R/IL-12RB2 genes appeared to be consistent in multiple reports with different populations including Turkey [52], Japanese [53], Han Chinese [62, 63], Iranian [64], Western Algeria [65], and Korean [66].

3.3 IL-33

IL-33 is a member of the IL-1 family that drives production of Th2-associated cytokines [67]. A small Iranian cohort of BD patients showed a significantly higher prevalence of the IL-33 SNP rs1342326T/G, and this genotype was also associated with higher IL-33 expression in the PBMC of the BD patients [68].

4. Genes involved in inflammation and autoimmunity

4.1 MEFV

The Mediterranean fever (MEFV) protein, also named pyrin is an important regulator of innate immunity [69]. Of noting, familial Mediterranean fever and BD share inflammatory nature and high prevalence in Middle Eastern and

Mediterranean populations. Genetically, the MEFV SNPs rs61752717 Met694Val, rs28940580 Met680Ile, and rs3743930 Glu148Gln confer risk to both diseases [61, 70–74]. Moreover, Met694Val and Met680Ile of the MEFV gene were also associated with greater responsiveness to bacterial products [72, 73].

4.2 IRF8

Interferon regulatory factor (IRF) 8 is a member of the interferon (IFN) regulatory factor (IRF) family, and it acts as a transcription factor to regulate the development and function of a variety of immune cells. In particular, it regulates expression of type I IFN stimulated genes [75], and interacts with the Th17 master transcription factor, ROR-γt to inhibit Th17 cell differentiation [76]. In a study with Chinese cohort, the IRF8 SNPs rs17445836 and rs11642873 were associated with BD, and they appeared to regulate IRF8 expression and corresponding cytokine production [77]. In another study with multiple cohorts including Turkish, Iranian, and Japanese patients, three other BD-associated SNPs (rs11117433, rs142105922 and rs7203487) of the IRF8 gene were reported [78].

4.3 TNFAIP3

TNF-α-induced protein 3 (TNFAIP3) is a ubiquitin-modifying enzyme A20 that regulates inflammation through NF-κB signaling pathway, and it can be induced by TNF, Toll-like receptors (TLRs), IL-1R, and NOD2 signaling [79–82]. The reports of genetic association between TNFAIP3 and BD appeared conflict in studies of Chinese and European populations. In the former, the TNFAIP3 SNPs (rs9494885, rs10499194 and rs7753873) were associated with BD [83], but were not replicated in the latter [84]. On the other hand, a Japanese study of familial BD indicated that a missense mutation C243Y in A20/TNFAIP3 was likely responsible for an increased production of some inflammatory cytokines by reduced suppression of NF-κB activation [85].

4.4 REL

The REL gene encodes for c-Rel, a member of the NF-κB family of transcription factors. It may play important roles in regulation of immune activity [86, 87]. A Chinese study indicated that the REL SNPs rs842647 may confer susceptibility to BD, and the allele C of this SNP was also associated with skin lesions in BD patients [88].

4.5 TLR2 and TLR4

Toll-like receptors (TLR) are transmembrane proteins that mediate innate immunity by recognizing pathogen molecules [89]. TLR2 and TLR4 are two members of the TLR, and they may transduce response to different types of pathogens (e.g., in macrophages, the former mainly for Gram-positive bacteria and the latter for Gram-negative). The TLR2 SNP rs2289318 (C allele and genotype CC) and rs3804099 (CT genotype) were associated with ocular BD in a Chinese cohort [90]. The associations of the TLR4 gene with BD are conflict in different reports. It was found in Japanese [91], Korea [92] and Turkish cohorts [66], but not in Italian [93], Tunisian [94], and Chinese cohorts [95]. Of note, two BD protective TLR4 variants identified in the Turkish cohort, p.Asp299Gly (rs4986790) and p.Thr399Ile (rs4986791) were associated with hyporesponsiveness to endotoxin [96].

4.6 NOD1 and NOD2

Nucleotide-binding oligomerization domain (NOD)-like receptors are intracellular proteins that regulate innate immune response. NOD1 and NOD2 proteins are two members of the NOD family, and they play important roles in initiating inflammation in response to microbial components [97, 98]. In a Chinese report, the minor allele (G) of the NOD1 SNP rs2075818 was protective from BD [35]. Multiple studies indicated that a Crohn's disease-associated polymorphism, Arg702Trp of the NOD2 rs2066844 was also protective from BD [61, 99, 100].

4.7 CCR1 and CCR3

CCR1 and CCR3 proteins are two C-C motif chemokine receptor (CCR) family members. They mediate signal transduction within cells in response to pathogens, and they are critical for the recruitment of effector immune cells to the site of inflammation, and for maintaining homeostasis of the immune system [101]. The CCR1 and 3 genes are clustered together on chromosome 3p. The Several SNPs at CCR1-CCR3 locus were associated with BD including rs7616215 in Turkish [40] and rs13084057, rs13092160 and rs13075270 in Chinese Cohorts [102]. In addition, the CCR1 gene was individually associated with BD in multiple cohorts including Turkish, Japanese, and Iranian cohorts [36, 103]. Functional studies indicated that CCR1 gene expression in primary human monocytes carrying the BD-risk allele was reduced along with a weaker activity of monocyte chemotaxis [36].

4.8 GIMAP

GTPase of the immunity-associated protein (GIMAP) family is a group of newly identified proteins. Although their functions are still poorly characterized, it is believed that they are lymphocyte signaling molecules, and they are also involved in survival and apoptosis of T cells and some other cell types [104, 105]. A GIMAP cluster including SNPs in GIMAP1 (rs2286900), GIMAP2 (rs10266069 and rs10256482), and GIMAP4 (rs1916012, rs1522596, and rs1608157) was associated with BD in a study of Korean and Japanese populations [106], but it failed in a replication study of European cohort [107].

4.9 KLRC4

Killer cell lectin-like receptor subfamily C, member 4 (KLRC4) is a member of NKG2 receptor family that regulates NK cell function. The association of the KLRC4 gene and BD was first suggested in the GWAS of Turkish and Japanese cohorts [36], and then replicated in the independent study of an Iranian cohort [103].

5. Genes involved in transcriptional activation of immune regulation

5.1 STAT4

Signal transducer and activator of transcription-4 (STAT4) is a transcription factor that activates gene expression involved in functional regulation and differentiation of T-helper cells, natural killer (NK) cells, mast cells, and dendritic cells [108]. It modulates differentiation of naïve T cells into Th1 and Th17 cells [56, 109, 110].

The association between the STAT4 gene and BD appeared to be consistent in multiple independent studies including Han Chinese [107], Korean, Turkish, and

Iranians [36, 103]. Functional studies indicated that the risk allele A of the STAT4 SNP rs897200 was correlated with the increased mRNA level of the STAT4 gene, and with the increased gene and protein expression of IL-17, as well as with BD patients who have a higher clinical severity score [111].

5.2 NCOA5

Nuclear receptor coactivator-5 (NCOA5) protein regulates nuclear receptor subfamily 1 group D member 2 (NR1D2) and estrogen receptor 1 and 2 (ESR1 and ESR2) [112, 113]. The NCOA5 gene SNP rs2903908 was associated with BD patients, especially those affected with genital ulceration and uveitis in the Finland and the Turkish cohorts [114].

5.3 FOXP3

FOXP3 (forkhead box P3), also known as scurfin, is a member of the FOX protein family of transcription factors. It regulates the development and function of T regulatory (Treg) cells [115, 116]. The FOXP3 SNP rs3761548 was associated with BD in the North-Western Iranian population [117]. In addition, a low copy number variant (CNV) of the FOXP3 gene was reported to confer risk to female BD patients in a Chinese cohort [118].

6. Other genes

6.1 PSORS1C1

Psoriasis susceptibility 1 candidate 1 (PSORS1C1) is poorly characterized in terms of its biological function. It is initially recognized as a susceptibility locus to psoriasis [119] and psoriatic arthritis [120]. Recent studies indicated that it is also a shared genetic factor, especially with SNP rs12525170, in other autoimmune diseases including systemic sclerosis [121], Crohn's disease [122], and BD [122]. Therefore, it may play important roles in the pathogenesis of autoimmunity [123, 124].

6.2 FUT2

Fucosyltransferase 2 (FUT2) is involved in synthesis of the H antigen, the precursor of the ABO-histo-blood group antigen in body fluids, and on the intestinal mucosa [125]. The association between the FUT2 gene (rs632111, rs601338, rs602662, rs492602, rs681343, and rs281377) and BD was reported in Iranian and Turkish populations [126].

6.3 UBAC2

Ubiquitin-associated domain containing 2 (UBAC2) is another poorly characterized protein, but its gene variants are strongly associated with BD. Limited studies suggest that it may function in protein localization in the endoplasmic reticulum [127]. The association of the UBAC2 gene with BD was found in Turkish, Chinese, Italian, and Japanese populations [128–131]. Functionally, the presence of BD-risk rs9517723 allele was correlated with an increased expression of the UBAC2 gene.

6.4 SUMO4

Small ubiquitin-like modifier 4 (SUMO4) is a member of the SUMO family that post-transcriptionally sumoylates the targeted proteins to regulate their subcellular localization and/or enhance their stability and activity [132]. It is involved in immune regulation by negatively controlling NFκB activity [133]. The genetic association between the SUMO4 (SNPs rs237024, rs237026) and BD was first reported in a Chinese cohort, and that appeared independent from HLA-B51 [134]. The association was replicated in Tunisian and Korean cohorts [135, 136], in which specific polymorphisms were also associated with disease severity, skin lesions, and vascular involvement of BD patients [135, 136].

6.5 LACC1

LACC1 encodes an oxidoreductase that promotes fatty-acid oxidation. It also functions in activation of inflammasome, bactericidal activity of macrophages, and production of mitochondrial and NADPH-oxidase-dependent reactive oxygen species [137]. SNP rs9316059 of the LACC1 was associated with BD in Turkish, Japanese, and Chinese cohorts [78, 138].

6.6 Loci at ADO-EGR2 and CEBPB-PTPN1

Two genetic loci between the ADO and the EGR2 genes and the CEBPB and the PTPN1 genes were associated with BD in the Turkish, Iranian, and Japanese cohorts [78]. The ADO encodes cysteamine (2-aminoethanethiol) dioxygenase that is involved in amino acid metabolism [139]. The EGR2 encodes early growth response protein 2 that is a transcription factor, and highly expressed in a population of migrating neural crest cells [140]. CEBPB encodes CCAAT/enhancer binding protein beta, a member of the CCAAT/enhancer binding protein family of basic leucine zipper transcription factors. It functions in controlling cell differentiation, proliferation, and inflammation [141]. The PTPN1 gene encodes protein tyrosine phosphatase, nonreceptor type 1 that functions as a key regulator of immune homeostasis by inhibiting T-cell receptor signaling and by selectively promoting type I interferon responses after activation of myeloid-cell pattern-recognition receptors [142].

It is worth noting that these BD-linked loci do not directly reflect the association of the corresponding genes, but may be suggestive for further investigation of these genes in terms of their genetic and functional importance to BD.

7. Conclusion

Multiple genes have been associated with BD, and many of them are involved in immune activation and regulation that may suggest their potential biological relevance to chronic inflammatory nature of BD. However, exact pathogenic mechanisms of BD on these genes are still unclear. Like many other immune-regulatory diseases, this multigenic feature of BD underlies complex pathogenesis. Some of the reported associations, for example, TNFAIP3 and TLR4, appeared to be conflict in different study cohorts and/or populations, which suggests that the BD-associated polymorphisms of the genes may be ethnic specific, or sample selection bias may have occurred and further verification may be warranted. In addition, some of the BD-associated genes, for example, HLA-B, ERAP1, MICA, and IL family, have also been reported in other immune-mediated diseases, which supports the shared genetic effects among these diseases. Moreover, specific gene polymorphisms were associated with clinical presentation of BD, for example, HLA-A02:07 with skin lesions and arthritis, HLA-A*26:01 with uveitis, HLA-A*30:04 with vascular lesions and genital ulcers, MICA-A5.1 with ocular lesions, and MICA-A9 with neurological and intestinal involvement. Thus, these specific genotypes may be further explored as potential biomarkers for diagnostic or prognostic classification of BD patients.

While the genetic studies have supported multigenic contribution to susceptibility to BD, epigenetic alternations including DNA methylation, histone modifications, and microRNAs regulation have also been reported in BD [143]. Furthermore, there is appealing evidence indicating environmental factors, especially that microorganisms may trigger the disease [144]. Understanding the genetics of BD in conjunction with epigenetics and environmental triggers of BD will provide insights into pathogenesis of the disease and an opportunity to interrogate candidate genes in potential diagnostic and therapeutic applications.

Author details

Xiaodong Zhou[1]* and Yan Deng[2]

1 Department of Internal Medicine/Rheumatology, University of Texas Health Science Center at Houston McGovern Medical School, USA

2 The Second Affiliated Hospital of Nanchang University, Nanchang, China

*Address all correspondence to: xiaodong.zhou@uth.tmc.edu and zhouxd@hotmail.com

References

[1] Saadoun D, Wechsler B. Behçet's disease. Orphanet Journal of Rare Diseases. 2012;**12**(7):20

[2] Verity DH, Marr JE, Ohno S, Wallace GR, Stanford MR. Behçet's disease, the silk road and HLA-B51: Historical and geographical perspectives. Tissue Antigens. 1999;**54**:213-220

[3] Calamia KT, Wilson FC, Icen M, Crowson CS, Gabriel SE, Kremers HM. HLA and non-HLA genes in Behçet's disease: A multicentric study in the Spanish population: A population-based study. Arthritis and Rheumatism. 2009;**61**:600-604

[4] Shahram F, Jamshidi AR, Hirbod-Mobarakeh A, Habibi G, Mardani A, Ghaemi M. Scientometric analysis and mapping of scientific articles on Behçet's disease. International Journal of Rheumatic Diseases. 2013;**16**:185-192

[5] Azizlerli G, Kose AA, Sarica R, Gul A, Tutkun IT, Kulac M, et al. Prevalence of Behçet's disease in Istanbul. Turkey International Journal of Dermatology. 2003;**42**:803-806

[6] Yurdakul S, Günaydin I, Tüzün Y, Tankurt N, Pazarli H, Ozyazgan Y, et al. The prevalence of Behçet's syndrome in a rural area in northern Turkey. The Journal of Rheumatology. 1988;**15**:820-822

[7] Idil A, Gurler A, Boyvat A, Caliskan D, Ozdemir O, Isik A, et al. The prevalence of Behçet's disease above the age of 10 years. The results of a pilot study conducted at the Park primary health care center in Ankara, Turkey. Ophthalmic Epidemiology. 2002;**9**:325-331

[8] Ozyurt K, Colgecen E, Baykan H. Does familial occurrence or family history of recurrent oral ulcers influence clinical characteristics of Behçet's disease? Acta Dermatovenerologica Croatica. 2013;**21**(3):168-173

[9] Davatchi F, Shahram F, Chams-Davatchi C, Sadeghi Abdollahi B, Shams H, Nadji A, et al. Behçet's disease: Is there a gender influence on clinical manifestations? International Journal of Rheumatic Diseases. 2012;**15**:306-314

[10] Ono S, Aoki K, Sugiura S, Nakayama E, Letter IK. HL-A5 and Behçet's disease. Lancet. 1973;**2**:1383-1384

[11] Ohno S, Ohguchi M, Hirose S, Matsuda H, Wakisaka A, Aizawa M. Close association of HLA-Bw51 with Behçet's disease. Archives of Ophthalmology. 1982;**100**:1455-1458

[12] Saadoun D, Wechsler B, Desseaux K, Le Thi Huong D, Amoura Z, Resche-Rigon M, et al. Mortality in Behçet's disease. Arthritis and Rheumatism. 2010;**62**:2806-2812

[13] Demirseren DD, Ceylan GG, Akoglu G, Emre S, Erten S, Arman A, et al. HLA-B51 subtypes in Turkish patients with Behçet's disease and their correlation with clinical manifestations. Genetics and Molecular Research. 2014;**13**:4788-4796

[14] Hamzaoui A, Houman MH, Massouadia M, Ben Salem T, Khanfir MS, Ben Ghorbel I, et al. Contribution of Hla-B51 in the susceptibility and specific clinical features of Behçet's disease in Tunisian patients. European Journal of Internal Medicine. 2012;**23**(4):347-349

[15] Salvarani C, Boiardi L, Mantovani V, Olivieri I, Ciancio G, Cantini F, et al. Association of MICA alleles and HLA-B51 in Italian patients with Behçet's disease. Journal of Rheumatology. 2001;**28**:1867-1870

[16] Kilmartin DJ, Finch A, Acheson RW. Primary association of HLA-B51 with Behçet's disease in Ireland. British Journal of Ophthalmology. 1997;**81**:649-653

[17] Lennikov A, Alekberova Z, Goloeva R, Kitaichi N, Denisov L, Namba K, et al. Single center study on ethnic and clinical features of Behçet's disease in Moscow, Russia. Clinical Rheumatology. 2015;**34**:321-327

[18] Paul M, Klein T, Krause I, Molad Y, Narinsky R, Weinberger A. Allelic distribution of HLA-B*5 in HLA-B5-positive Israeli patients with Behçet's disease. Tissue Antigens. 2001;**58**:185-186

[19] Mizuki N, Ota M, Katsuyama Y, Yabuki K, Ando H, Shiina T, et al. Sequencing-based typing of HLA-B*51 alleles and the significant association of HLA-B*5101 and -B*5108 with Behçet's disease in Greek patients. Tissue Antigens. 2002;**59**:118-121

[20] Koumantaki Y, Stavropoulos C, Spyropoulou M, Messini H, Papademetropoulos M, Giziaki E, et al. HLA-B5101 in Greek patients with Behçet's disease. Human Immunology. 1998;**59**:250-255

[21] Mizuki N, Ota M, Katsuyama Y, Yabuki K, Ando H, Yoshida M, et al. HLA class I genotyping including HLA-B*51 allele typing in the Iranian patients with Behçet's disease. Tissue Antigens. 2001;**57**:457-462

[22] Ortiz-Fernández L, Carmona FD, Montes-Cano MA, García-Lozano JR, Conde-Jaldón M, Ortego-Centeno N, et al. Genetic analysis with the immunochip platform in Behçet disease. Identification of residues associated in the HLA Class I region and new susceptibility loci. PLoS One. 2016;**11**:e0161305

[23] de Menthon M, Lavalley MP, Maldini C, Guillevin L, Mahr A. HLA-B51/B5 and the risk of Behçet's disease: A systematic review and meta-analysis of case-control genetic association studies. Arthritis and Rheumatism. 2009;**61**:1287-1296

[24] Montes-Cano MA, Conde-Jaldón M, García-Lozano JR, et al. HLA and non-HLA genes in Behçet's disease: A multicentric study in the Spanish population. Arthritis Research & Therapy. 2013;**15**:145

[25] Takeuchi M, Kastner DL, Remmers EF. The immunogenetics of Behçet's disease: A comprehensive review. Journal of Autoimmunity. 2015;**64**:137-148

[26] Radouane A, Oudghiri M, Chakib A, Naya A, Belhouari A, El Malki A, et al. HLA-B*27 allele associated to Behçet's disease and to anterior uveitis in Moroccan patients. Annales de Biologie Clinique. 2011;**69**:419-424

[27] Al Mosawi ZS, Madan W, Fareed E. Pediatric-onset Behçet disease in Bahrain: Report of nine cases and literature review. Archives of Iranian Medicine. 2012;**15**(8):485-487

[28] Meguro A, Inoko H, Ota M, Katsuyama Y, Oka A, Okada E, et al. Genetics of Behçet disease inside and outside the MHC. Annals of the Rheumatic Diseases. 2010;**69**:747-754

[29] Al-Okaily F, Al-Rashidi S, Al-Balawi M, Mustafa M, Arfin M, Al-Asmari A. Genetic association of HLA-A*26, -A*31, and -B*51 with Behçet's disease in Saudi patients. Clinical Medicine Insights: Arthritis and Musculoskeletal Disorders. 2016;**9**:167-173

[30] Kaburaki T, Takamoto M, Numaga J, Kawashima H, Araie M, Ohnogi Y, et al. Genetic association of HLA-A*2601 with ocular Behçet's disease in Japanese patients. Clinical and Experimental Rheumatology. 2010;**28**:S39-S44

[31] Kang EH, Park JW, Park C, Yu HG, Lee EB, Park MH, et al. Genetic and non-genetic factors affecting the visual outcome of ocular Behçet's disease. Human Immunology. 2013;**74**:1363-1367

[32] Kang EH, Kim JY, Takeuchi F, Kim JW, Shin K, Lee EY, et al. Associations between the HLA-A polymorphism and the clinical manifestations of Behçet's disease. Arthritis Research & Therapy. 2011;**13**:R49

[33] Ting JP, Trowsdale J. Genetic control of MHC class II expression. Cell. 2002;**109**:S21-S33

[34] Devaiah BN, Singer DS. CIITA and its dual roles in MHC gene transcription. Frontiers in Immunology. 2013;**4**:476-481

[35] Li L, Yu H, Jiang Y, Deng B, Bai L, Kijlstra A, et al. Genetic variations of NLR family genes in Behçet's disease. Scientific Reports. 2016;**6**:20098-20104

[36] Kirino Y, Bertsias G, Ishigatsubo Y, et al. Genome-wide association analysis identifies new susceptibility loci for Behçet's disease and epistasis between HLA-B*51 and ERAP1. Nature Genetics. 2013;**45**:202-207

[37] Zhang L, Yu H, Zheng M, Li H, Liu Y, Kijlstra A, et al. Association of ERAP1 gene polymorphisms with Behçet's disease in Han Chinese. Investigative Ophthalmology & Visual Science. 2015;**56**:6029-6035

[38] Conde-Jaldón M, Montes-Cano MA, García-Lozano JR, Ortiz-Fernández L, Ortego-Centeno N, González-León R, et al. Epistatic interaction of ERAP1 and HLA-B in Behçet disease: A replication study in the Spanish population. PLoS One. 2014;**9**:e102100

[39] Choy MK, Phipps ME. MICA polymorphism: Biology and importance in immunity and disease. Trends in Molecular Medicine. 2010;**16**:97-106

[40] Bahram S, Bresnahan M, Geraghty DE, Spies T. A second lineage of mammalian major histocompatibility complex class I genes. Proceedings of the National Academy of Sciences of the United States of America. 1994;**91**:6259-6263

[41] Zhou X, Wang J, Zou H, Ward MM, Weisman MH, Espitia MG, et al. MICA, a gene contributing strong susceptibility to ankylosing spondylitis. Annals of the Rheumatic Diseases. 2014;**73**:1552-1557

[42] Muñoz-Saá I, Cambra A, Pallarés L, Espinosa G, Juan A, Pujalte F, et al. Allelic diversity and affinity variants of MICA are imbalanced in Spanish patients with Behçet's disease. Scandinavian Journal of Immunology. 2006;**64**:77-82

[43] Mizuki N, Ota M, Kimura M, Ohno S, Ando H, Katsuyama Y, et al. Triplet repeat polymorphism in the transmembrane region of the MICA gene: A strong association of six GCT repetitions with Behçet disease. Proceedings of the National Academy of Sciences of the United States of America. 1997;**94**:1298-1303

[44] Wei F, Zhang YU, Li W. A meta-analysis of the association between Behçet's disease and MICA-A6. Biomedical Reports. 2016;**4**:741-745

[45] Park SH, Park KS, Seo YI, Min DJ, Kim WU, Kim TG, et al. Association of MICA polymorphism with HLA-B51 and disease severity in Korean patients with Behçet's disease. Journal of Korean Medical Science. 2002;**17**:366-370

[46] Zhang J, Liao D, Yang L, Hou S. Association between Functional MICA-TM and Behçet's disease: A systematic review and meta-analysis. Scientific Reports. 2016;**6**:21033

[47] Nishiyama M, Takahashi M, Kuriyama T, Nakae K. Research report: Frequencies of mica gene

polymorphism: A comparison between Indonesians on Bacan Island and suburban Japanese. The Southeast Asian Journal of Tropical Medicine and Public Health. 2004;**35**:195-201

[48] Fiorentino DF, Zlotnik A, Vieira P, Mosmann TR, Howard M, Moore KW, et al. IL-10 acts on the antigen-presenting cell to inhibit cytokine production by Th1 cells. Journal of Immunology. 1991;**146**:3444-3451

[49] Mosmann TR, Coffman RL. TH1 and TH2 cells: Different patterns of lymphokine secretion lead to different functional properties. Annual Review of Immunology. 1989;**7**:145-173

[50] Wallace GR, Kondeatis E, Vaughan RW, et al. IL-10 genotype analysis in patients with Behçet's disease. Human Immunology. 2007;**68**:122-127

[51] Hu J, Hou S, Zhu X, Fang J, Zhou Y, Liu Y, et al. Interleukin-10 gene polymorphisms are associated with Behçet's disease but not with Vogt-Koyanagi-Harada syndrome in the Chinese Han population. Molecular Vision. 2015;**21**:589-603

[52] Remmers EF, Cosan F, Kirino Y, et al. Genome-wide association study identifies variants in the MHC class I, IL10, and IL23R-IL12RB2 regions associated with Behçet's disease. Nature Genetics. 2010;**42**:698-702

[53] Mizuki N, Meguro A, Ota M, Ohno S, Shiota T, Kawagoe T, et al. Genome-wide association studies identify IL23R-IL12RB2 and IL10 as Behçet's disease susceptibility loci. Nature Genetics. 2010;**42**:703-706

[54] Akdis M, Burgler S, Crameri R, et al. Interleukins, from 1 to 37, and interferon-γ: Receptors, functions, and roles in diseases. The Journal of Allergy and Clinical Immunology. 2011;**127**:701-721

[55] Chang JT, Shevach EM, Segal BM. Regulation of interleukin (IL)-12 receptor beta2 subunit expression by endogenous IL-12: A critical step in the differentiation of pathogenic autoreactive T cells. The Journal of Experimental Medicine. 1999;**189**:969-978

[56] Watford WT, Hissong BD, Bream JH, et al. Signaling by IL-12 and IL-23 and the immunoregulatory roles of STAT4. Immunological Reviews. 2004;**202**:139-156

[57] Kappen JH, Medina-Gomez C, van Hagen PM, et al. Genome-wide association study in an admixed case series reveals IL12A as a new candidate in Behçet disease. PLoS One. 2015;**10**:e0119085

[58] Murphy CA, Langrish CL, Chen Y, et al. Divergent pro-and antiinflammatory roles for IL-23 and IL-12 in joint autoimmune inflammation. The Journal of Experimental Medicine. 2003;**198**:1951-1957

[59] Iwakura Y, Ishigame H. The IL-23/IL-17 axis in inflammation. The Journal of Clinical Investigation. 2006;**116**:1218-1222

[60] Steinman L. Mixed results with modulation of TH-17 cells in human autoimmune diseases. Nature Immunology. 2010;**11**:41-44

[61] Kirino Y, Zhou Q, Ishigatsubo Y, Mizuki N, Tugal-Tutkun I, Seyahi E, et al. Targeted resequencing implicates the familial Mediterranean fever gene MEFV and the toll-like receptor 4 gene TLR4 in Behçet disease. Proceedings of the National Academy of Sciences of the United States of America. 2013;**110**:8134-8139

[62] Yu H, Zheng M, Zhang L, Li H, Zhu Y, Cheng L, et al. Identification of susceptibility SNPs in IL10 and IL23R-IL12RB2 for Behçet's disease in Han

Chinese. The Journal of Allergy and Clinical Immunology. 2017;**139**:621-627

[63] Qin X, Xu J, Wu Z, Sun F, Chen H, Zheng W, et al. Association study of rs924080 and rs11209032 polymorphisms of IL23R-IL12RB2 in a northern Chinese Han population with Behçet's disease. Human Immunology. 2016;**77**:1284-1290

[64] Xavier JM, Shahram F, Davatchi F, et al. Association study of IL10 and IL23R-IL12RB2 in Iranian patients with Behçet's disease. Arthritis and Rheumatism. 2012;**64**:2761-2772

[65] Khaib Dit Naib O, Aribi M, Idder A, Chiali A, Sairi H, Touitou I, et al. Association analysis of IL10, TNF-α, and IL23R-IL12RB2 SNPs with Behçet's disease risk in Western Algeria. Frontiers in Immunology. 2013;**4**:342

[66] Kang EH, Kim S, Park MY, Choi JY, Choi IA, Kim MJ, et al. Behçet's disease risk association fine-mapped on the IL23R-IL12RB2 intergenic region in Koreans. Arthritis Research & Therapy. 2017;**19**:227

[67] Mirchandani AS, Salmond RJ, Liew FY. Interleukin-33 and the function of innate lymphoid cells. Trends in Immunology. 2012;**33**(8):389-396

[68] Talei M, Abdi A, Shanebandi D, Jadidi-Niaragh F, Khabazi A, Babaie F, et al. Interleukin-33 gene expression and rs1342326 polymorphism in Behçet's disease. Immunology Letters. 2018;**S0165-2478**(17):30443-30441

[69] Chae JJ, Wood G, Masters SL, Richard K, Park G, Smith BJ, et al. The B30.2 domain of pyrin, the familial Mediterranean fever protein, interacts directly with caspase-1 to modulate IL-1beta production. Proceedings of the National Academy of Sciences of the United States of America. 2006;**103**:9982-9987

[70] French FMF Consortium. A candidate gene for familial Mediterranean fever. Nature Genetics. 1997;**17**:25-31

[71] Touitou I, Magne X, Molinari N, Navarro A, Quellec AL, et al. MEFV mutations in Behçet's disease. Human Mutation. 2000;**16**:271-272

[72] Esmaeili M, Bonyadi M, Khabbazi A, Ebrahimi AA, Sharif SK, et al. Common MEFV mutations in Iranian Azeri Turkish patients with Behçet's disease. Scandinavian Journal of Rheumatology. 2011;**40**:383-386

[73] Wu Z, Zhang S, Li J, Chen S, Li P, Sun F, et al. Association between MEFV mutations M694V and M680I and Behçet's disease: A meta-analysis. PLoS One. 2015;**10**:e0132704

[74] Tasliyurt T, Yigit S, Rustemoglu A, Gul U, Ates O. Common MEFV gene mutations in Turkish patients with Behçet's disease. Gene. 2013;**530**:100-103

[75] Holtschke T, Lohler J, Kanno Y, Fehr T, Giese N, Rosenbauer F, et al. Immunodeficiency and chronic myelogenous leukemia-like syndrome in mice with a targeted mutation of the ICSBP gene. Cell. 1996;**87**:307-317

[76] Ouyang X, Zhang R, Yang J, Li Q, Qin L, Zhu C, et al. Transcription factor IRF8 directs a silencing programme for TH17 cell differentiation. Nature Communications. 2011;**2**:314

[77] Jiang Y, Wang H, Yu H, Li L, Xu D, Hou S, et al. Two genetic variations in the IRF8 region are associated with Behçet's disease in Han Chinese. Scientific Reports. 2016;**6**:19651

[78] Takeuchi M, Mizuki N, Meguro A, Ombrello MJ, Kirino Y, Satorius C, et al. Dense genotyping of immune-related loci implicates host responses to microbial exposure in Behçet's

disease susceptibility. Nature Genetics. 2017;**49**:438-443

[79] Boone DL, Turer EE, Lee EG, Ahmad RC, Wheeler MT, Tsui C, et al. The ubiquitin-modifying enzyme A20 is required for termination of toll-like receptor responses. Nature Immunology. 2004;**5**:1052-1060

[80] Hitotsumatsu O, Ahmad RC, Tavares R, Wang M, Philpott D, Turer EE, et al. The ubiquitin-editing enzyme A20 restricts nucleotide-binding oligomerization domain containing 2-triggered signals. Immunity. 2008;**28**:381-390

[81] Jaattela M, Mouritzen H, Elling F, Bastholm L. A20 zinc finger protein inhibits TNF and IL-1 signaling. Journal of Immunology. 1996;**156**:1166-1173

[82] Lee EG, Boone DL, Chai S, Libby SL, Chien M, Lodolce JP, et al. Failure to regulate TNF-induced NF-kappaB and cell death responses in A20-deficient mice. Science. 2000;**289**:2350-2354

[83] Li H, Liu Q, Hou S, Du L, Zhou Q, Zhou Y, et al. TNFAIP3 gene polymorphisms confer risk for Behçet's disease in a Chinese Han population. Human Genetics. 2013;**132**:293-300

[84] Ortiz-Fernández L, García-Lozano JR, Montes-Cano MA, Conde-Jaldón M, Ortego-Centeno N, et al. Lack of association of TNFAIP3 and JAK1 with Behçet's disease in the European population. Clinical and Experimental Rheumatology. 2015;**33**(6 Suppl 94): S36-S39

[85] Shigemura T, Kaneko N, Kobayashi N, Kobayashi K, Takeuchi Y, Nakano N, et al. Novel heterozygous C243Y A20/TNFAIP3 gene mutation is responsible for chronic inflammation in autosomal-dominant Behçet's disease. RMD Open. 2016;**2**:e000223

[86] Chen G, Hardy K, Pagler E, Ma L, Lee S, Gerondakis S, et al. The NF-κB transcription factor c-Rel is required for Th17 effector cell development in experimental autoimmune ncephalomyelitis. Journal of Immunology. 2011;**187**:4483-4491

[87] Lamhamedi-Cherradi SE, Zheng S, Hilliard BA, Xu L, Sun J, Alsheadat S, et al. Transcriptional regulation of type I diabetes by NF-kappa B. Journal of Immunology. 2003;**171**:4886-4892

[88] Chen F, Xu L, Zhao T, Xiao X, Pan Y, Hou S. Genetic variation in the REL gene increases risk of Behçet's disease in a Chinese Han population but that of PRKCQ does not. PLoS One. 2016;**11**:147350

[89] Poltorak A, He X, Smirnova I, Liu MY, Van Huffel C, Du X, et al. Defective LPS signaling in C3H/HeJ and C57BL/10ScCr mice: Mutations in Tlr4 gene. Science. 1998;**282**:2085-2088

[90] Fang J, Hu R, Hou S, Ye Z, Xiang Q, Qi J, et al. Association of TLR2 gene polymorphisms with ocular Behçet's disease in a Chinese Han population. Investigative Ophthalmology & Visual Science. 2013;**54**:8384-8392

[91] Meguro A, Ota M, Katsuyama Y, Oka A, Ohno S, Inoko H, et al. Association of the toll-like receptor 4 gene polymorphisms with Behçet's disease. Annals of the Rheumatic Diseases. 2008;**67**:725-727

[92] Horie Y, Meguro A, Ota M, Kitaichi N, Katsuyama Y, et al. Association of TLR4 polymorphisms with Behçet's disease in a Korean population. Rheumatology. 2009;**48**:638-642

[93] Boiardi L, Atzeni F, Casali B, Farnetti E, Nicoli D, et al. Toll-like receptor 4 (TLR4) gene polymorphisms in Italian patients with Behçet's disease. Clinical and Experimental Rheumatology. 2009;**27**(Suppl 53):S43-S47

[94] Ben Dhifallah I, Lachheb J, Houman H, Hamzaoui K. Toll-like-receptor gene polymorphisms in a Tunisian population with Behçet's disease. Clinical and Experimental Rheumatology. 2009;**27**(Suppl 53): S58-S62

[95] Du L, Yang P, Hou S, Zhou H, Kijlstra A. No association of CTLA-4 polymorphisms with susceptibility to Behçet disease. The British Journal of Ophthalmology. 2009;**93**:1378-1381

[96] Arbour NC, Lorenz E, Schutte BC, Zabner J, Kline JN, Jones M, et al. TLR4 mutations are associated with endotoxin hyporesponsiveness in humans. Nature Genetics. 2000;**25**:187-191

[97] Strober W, Murray PJ, Kitani A, Watanabe T. Signalling pathways and molecular interactions of NOD1 and NOD2. Nature Reviews Immunology. 2006;**6**:9-20

[98] Moreira LO, Zamboni DS. NOD1 and NOD2 signaling in infection and inflammation. Frontiers in Immunology. 2012;**3**:328-334

[99] Kappen JH, Wallace GR, Stolk L, Rivadeneira F, Uitterlinden AG, van Daele PL, et al. Low prevalence of NOD2 SNPs in Behçet's disease suggests protective association in Caucasians. Rheumatology. 2009;**48**:1375-1377

[100] Burillo-Sanz S, Montes-Cano MA, García-Lozano JR, Ortiz-Fernández L, Ortego-Centeno N. Mutational profile of rare variants in inflammasome-related genes in Behçet disease: A next generation sequencing approach. Scientific Reports. 2017;7:8453

[101] Di Marzio P, Dai WW, Franchin G, Chan AY, Symons M, Sherry B. Role of rho family GTPases in CCR1- and CCR5-induced actin reorganization in macrophages. Biochemical and Biophysical Research Communications. 2005;**331**:909-916

[102] Hou S, Xiao X, Li F, Jiang Z, Kijlstra A, Yang P. Two-stage association study in Chinese Han identifies two independent associations in CCR1/CCR3 locus as candidate for Behçet's disease susceptibility. Human Genetics. 2012;**131**:1841-1850

[103] Sousa I, Shahram F, Francisco D, Davatchi F, Abdollahi BS, Ghaderibarmi F, et al. Brief report: Association of CCR1, KLRC4, IL12A-AS1, STAT4, and ERAP1 with Behçet's disease in Iranians. Arthritis & Rhematology. 2015;**67**:2742-2748

[104] Filén JJ, Filén S, Moulder R, Tuomela S, Ahlfors H, West A, et al. Quantitative proteomics reveals GIMAP family proteins 1 and 4 to be differentially regulated during human T helper cell differentiation. Molecular & Cellular Proteomics. 2009;**8**:32-44

[105] Saunders A, Webb LM, Janas ML, Hutchings A, Pascall J, Carter C, et al. Putative GTPase GIMAP1 is critical for the development of mature B and T lymphocytes. Blood. 2010;**115**:3249-3257

[106] Lee YJ, Horie Y, Wallace GR, Choi YS, Park JA, Choi JY, et al. Genome-wide association study identifies GIMAP as a novel susceptibility locus for Behçet's disease. Annals of the Rheumatic Diseases. 2013;**72**:1510-1516

[107] Ortiz-Fernández L, Conde-Jaldón M, García-Lozano JR, Montes-Cano MA, Ortego-Centeno N, Castillo-Palma MJ, et al. GIMAP and Behçet disease: no association in the European population. Annals of the Rheumatic Diseases. 2014;**73**:1433-1454

[108] Morinobu A, Gadina M, Strober W, Visconti R, Fornace A, Montagna C, et al. STAT4 serine phosphorylation is critical for IL-12-induced IFN-gamma production but not for cell proliferation. Proceedings of the National Academy

of Sciences of the United States of America. 2002;**99**:12281-12286

[109] Kim J, Park JA, Lee EY, Lee YJ, Song YW, Lee EB. Imbalance of Th17 to Th1 cells in Behçet's disease. Clinical and Experimental Rheumatology. 2010;**28**:S16-S19

[110] Mathur AN, Chang HC, Zisoulis DG, Stritesky GL, Yu Q, O'Malley JT, et al. Stat3 and Stat4 direct development of IL-17-secreting Th cells. Journal of Immunology. 2007;**178**:4901-4907

[111] Hou S, Yang Z, Du L, Jiang Z, Shu Q, Chen Y, et al. Identification of a susceptibility locus in STAT4 for Behçet's disease in Han Chinese in a genome-wide association study. Arthritis and Rheumatism. 2012;**64**:4104-4113

[112] Zervou MI, Goulielmos GN, Castro-Giner F, Boumpas DT, Tosca AD, Krueger-Krasagakis S. A CD40 and an NCOA5 gene polymorphism confer susceptibility to psoriasis in a southern European population: A case-control study. Human Immunology. 2011;**72**:761-765

[113] Böser A, Drexler HC, Reuter H, Schmitz H, Wu G, Schöler HR, et al. SILAC proteomics of planarians identifies NCOA5 as a conserved component of pluripotent stem cells. Cell Reports. 2013;**5**:1142-1155

[114] Rustemoglu A, Erkol Inal E, Inanir A, Ekinci D, Gul U, Yigit S, et al. Clinical significance of NCOA5 gene rs2903908 polymorphism in Behçet's disease. EXCLI Journal. 2017;**16**:609-617

[115] Fontenot JD, Rasmussen JP, Williams LM, Dooley JL, Farr AG, Rudensky AY. Regulatory T cell lineage specification by the forkhead transcription factor foxp3. Immunity. 2005;**22**(3):329-341

[116] Marson A, Kretschmer K, Frampton GM, Jacobsen ES, Polansky JK, MacIsaac KD, et al. Foxp3 occupancy and regulation of key target genes during T-cell stimulation. Nature. 2007;**445**(7130):931-935

[117] Hosseini A, Shanehbandi D, Estiar MA, Gholizadeh S, Khabbazi A, Khodadadi H, et al. A single nucleotide polymorphism in the FOXP3 gene associated with Behçet's disease in an Iranian population. Clinical Laboratory. 2015;**61**(12):1897-1903

[118] Liao D, Hou S, Zhang J, Fang J, Liu Y, Bai L, et al. Copy number variants and genetic polymorphisms in TBX21, GATA3, Rorc, Foxp3 and susceptibility to Behçet's disease and Vogt-Koyanagi-Harada syndrome. Scientific Reports. 2015;**5**:9511

[119] Holm SJ, Carlén LM, Mallbris L, Ståhle-Bäckdahl M, O'Brien KP. Polymorphisms in the SEEK1 and SPR1 genes on 6p21.3 associate with psoriasis in the Swedish population. Experimental Dermatology. 2003;**12**:435-444

[120] Rahman P, Butt C, Siannis F, Farewell VT, Peddle L, Pellett FJ, et al. Association of SEEK1 and psoriatic arthritis in two distinct Canadian populations. Annals of the Rheumatic Diseases. 2005;**64**:1370-1372

[121] Bossini-Castillo L, Martin JE, Broen J, Simeon CP, Beretta L, Gorlova OY, et al. Confirmation of TNIP1 but not RHOB and PSORS1C1 as systemic sclerosis risk factors in a large independent replication study. Annals of the Rheumatic Diseases. 2013;**72**:602-607

[122] Peddle L, Zipperlen K, Melay B, Hefferton D, Rahman P. Association of SEEK1 polymorphisms in Crohn's disease. Human Immunology. 2004;**65**:706-709

[123] Fan X, Yang S, Huang W, Wang ZM, Sun LD, Liang YH, et al. Fine

mapping of the psoriasis susceptibility locus PSORS1 supports HLA-C as the susceptibility gene in the Han Chinese population. PLoS Genetics. 2008;**4**:e1000038

[124] Reich K, Hüffmeier U, König IR, Lascorz J, Lohmann J, Wendler J, et al. TNF polymorphisms in psoriasis: Association of psoriatic arthritis with the promoter polymorphism TNF*-857 independent of the PSORS1 risk allele. Arthritis and Rheumatism. 2007;**56**:2056-2064

[125] Ferrer-Admetlla A, Sikora M, Laayouni H, Esteve A, Roubinet F, Blancher A, et al. A natural history of FUT2 polymorphism in humans. Molecular Biology and Evolution. 2009;**26**:1993-2003

[126] Xavier JM, Shahram F, Sousa I, Davatchi F, Matos M, Abdollahi BS, et al. FUT2: Filling the gap between genes and environment in Behçet's disease? Annals of the Rheumatic Diseases. 2015;**74**:618-624

[127] Olzmann JA, Richter CM, Kopito RR. Spatial regulation of UBXD8 and p97/VCP controls ATGL-mediated lipid droplet turnover. Proceedings of the National Academy of Sciences of the United States of America. 2013;**110**:1345-1350

[128] Fei Y, Webb R, Cobb BL, Direskeneli H, Saruhan-Direskeneli G, Sawalha AH. Identification of novel genetic susceptibility loci for Behçet's disease using a genome-wide association study. Arthritis Research & Therapy. 2009;**11**:R66

[129] Sawalha AH, Hughes T, Nadig A, Yılmaz V, Aksu K, Keser G, et al. A putative functional variant within the UBAC2 gene is associated with increased risk of Behçet's disease. Arthritis and Rheumatism. 2011;**63**:3607-3612

[130] Hou S, Shu Q, Jiang Z, Chen Y, Li F, Chen F, et al. Replication study confirms the association between UBAC2 and Behçet's disease in two independent Chinese sets of patients and controls. Arthritis Research & Therapy. 2012;**14**:R70

[131] Yamazoe K, Meguro A, Takeuchi M, Shibuya E, Ohno S, Mizuki N. Comprehensive analysis of the association between UBAC2 polymorphisms and Behçet's disease in a Japanese population. Scientific Reports. 2017;**7**:742-747

[132] Rallabhandi P, Hashimoto K, Mo YY, Beck WT, Moitra PK, D'Arpa P. Sumoylation of topoisomerase I is involved in its partitioning between nucleoli and nucleoplasm and its clearing from nucleoli in response to camptothecin. The Journal of Biological Chemistry. 2002;**277**:40020-40026

[133] Guo D, Li M, Zhang Y, Yang P, Eckenrode S, Hopkins D, et al. A functional variant of SUMO4, a new I kappa B alpha modifier, is associated with type 1 diabetes. Nature Genetics. 2004;**36**:837-841

[134] Hou S, Yang P, Du L, Zhou H, Lin X, Liu X, et al. SUMO4 gene polymorphisms in Chinese Han patients with Behçet's disease. Clinical Immunology. 2008;**129**:170-175

[135] Kamoun M, Ben Dhifallah I, Karray E, Zakraoui L, Hamzaoui K. Association of small ubiquitin-like modifier 4 (SUMO4) polymorphisms in a Tunisian population with Behçet's disease. Clinical and Experimental Rheumatology. 2010;**28**(Suppl. 60):S45-S49

[136] Park G, Kim HS, Choe JY, Kim SK. SUMO4 C438T polymorphism is associated with papulopustular skin lesion in Korean patients with Behçet's disease. Rheumatology International. 2012;**32**:3031-3037

[137] Cader MZ, Boroviak K, Zhang Q, Assadi G, Kempster SL, Sewell GW,

et al. C13orf31 (FAMIN) is a central regulator of immunometabolic function. Nature Immunology. 2016;**17**:1046-1056

[138] Wu P, Du L, Hou S, Su G, Yang L, Hu J, et al. Association of LACC1, CEBPB-PTPN1, RIPK2 and ADO-EGR2 with ocular Behçet's disease in a Chinese Han population. The British Journal of Ophthalmology. 2018;**102**:1308-1314

[139] Sarkar B, Kulharia M, Mantha AK. Understanding human thiol dioxygenase enzymes: Structure to function, and biology to pathology. International Journal of Experimental Pathology. 2017;**98**:52-66

[140] Wilkinson DG, Bhatt S, Chavrier P, et al. Segment-specific expression of a zinc-finger gene in the developing nervous system of the mouse. Nature. 1989;**337**(6206):461-464

[141] Nerlov C. The C/EBP family of transcription factors: A paradigm for interaction between gene expression and proliferation control. Trends in Cell Biology. 2007;**17**:318-324

[142] Sanford SM, Bottini N. PTPN22: The archetypal non-HLA autoimmunity gene. Nature Reviews Rheumatology. 2014;**10**:602-611

[143] Alipour S, Nouri M, Sakhinia E, Samadi N, Roshanravan N, Ghavami A, et al. Epigenetic alterations in chronic disease focusing on Behçet's disease: Review. Biomedicine & Pharmacotherapy. 2017;**91**:526-533

[144] Hatemi G, Yazici H. Behçet's syndrome and micro-organisms. Best Practice & Research. Clinical Rheumatology. 2011;**25**:389-406

Chapter 4

The Role of Th17 Cells in the Pathogenesis of Behçet's Disease

Yuki Nanke and Shigeru Kotake

Abstract

Behçet's disease (BD) is a polysymptomatic and recurrent systemic vasculitis with a chronic course and unknown cause. BD is now categorized as both autoimmune diseases and auto inflammatory diseases. The pathogenesis of BD is still unclear; however, BD has been thought as a Th1-related disease, with elevating levels of Th1 cytokines such as IFN-γ, TNF-α, and IL-2. Some investigators found that Th17-associated cytokines were elevated in patients with BD; thus, IL-17/IL-23 pathway and Th17 cells may have crucial roles in the pathogenesis of BD. In this chapter, we review the pathogenic role of Th17 cells in BD.

Keywords: IL-17, Th17, Th1, Behçet's disease, regulatory T cells

1. Introduction

BD is a systemic vasculitis and polysymptomatic [1, 2] and characterized by recurrent aphthous stomatitis, genital ulcers, uveitis, and skin lesions. Arthritis is also a common manifestation of BD, and sometimes inflammation is involved in the gastrointestinal tract as well as vascular and central nervous systems. The cause of BD is not fully understood. BD is now categorized as both an autoimmune disease and an autoinflammatory disease.

The association between carriage of the human leukocyte antigen (HLA) B51 allele and BD has been known in different ethnic groups. Recently, the genome-wide studies showed the association of some non-histocompatibility complex (MHC) genes, including IL-23R-IL-12 RB 2 and IL-10 genes [3, 4]. The pathogenesis of BD has not been fully elucidated; in addition to genetic factors, cytokines, viral and bacterial agents, and immune dysfunction are associated with the exacerbation of BD.

CD4+ T cells and neutrophils play an important role in the pathogenesis of BD. Since IL-12 and IFN-γ from Th1 cells can mediate the inflammatory response between neutrophils and T cells, BD has been considered as a Th1-mediated disease [5, 6].

Th17 cells play an important role in immunity. Th17 cell differentiation from naïve CD4+ T cells is assisted by IL-6, IL-21, IL-1β, and IL-23. The critical feature of Th17 cells is the expression of IL-17A, IL-17F, IL-22, IL-6, IL-8, and IL-26, and TNF-α expresses RAR-related orphan receptor (ROR) γ. The current studies suggest that Th17 axis plays a pivotal role in BD pathogenesis. IL-17 has been shown to recruit neutrophils to the site of inflammation. Abnormalities in the T cell response cause the hyperreactivity of neutrophils in BD through the production of cytokines, such as IL-17 [7]. We discuss the pathogenic role of Th17 cells in BD.

IntechOpen

2. Th17 in mouse model

In mice, the combination of IL-6 and TGF-β plays a critical role in the development of Th17 cells from naive T cells. Th17 cells play important roles in the pathogenesis of intraocular inflammation in an animal model of uveitis [8–10]. Anti-mouse IL-17 blocking antibodies are effective for intraocular inflammation in experimental models of uveitis [11].

Inhibition of the expression of TNF-α [12], and the downregulation of IL-6 [13] improved the inflammation in BD mice by the upregulation of Th17 cells. Foxp3 may inhibit Th17 differentiation by antagonizing the function of RORγt, the master transcription factor. It is reported that anti-TNF-α blockade may prevent the differentiation of Th17 cells in animal models for BD [14]. γδ T cells produce IL-17 and may play an important role in experimental uveitis in animal models [10].

3. Th17 in humans

3.1 Plasma IL-17 levels in BD

In humans, IL-23 and IL-1β are needed for the development of Th17 cells. IL-17 levels were markedly elevated in BD [15–20]. Some investigators [22, 23] reported that the ability to produce IL-17A and amount of circulating Th17 cells were increased in active BD patients. Increased levels of IL-17 may induce neutrophil activity [22].

It is reported that the ability to produce IL-17A and population of Th17 cells are enhanced in active BD despite the low expression of RORγt mRNA [21]. Chi et al. reported that elevated levels of IL-17A, IL-23, and IFN-γ in the aqueous fluid from the eyes as well as in peripheral blood of BD patients [23, 24].

3.2 Circulating Th17 cell frequencies are correlated with disease activity

It is reported that the significantly higher frequency of circulating Th17 cells are detected in active BD patients compared with the same patients in remission stages [21]. A positive correlation was seen between the plasma IL-17 level and ESR or CRP in active BD patients [21]. It has been reported that the peripheral blood Th17/Th1 ratio was markedly higher in patients with active BD than the healthy controls [25, 26] and that in BD patients with folliculitis or uveitis, the Th17/Th1 ratio was elevated [23, 24]. Thus, the balance of Th1 and Th17 cells plays an important role in the pathogenesis of BD, especially in the pathogenesis of folliculitis and uveitis. Moreover, the high expression of IL-23p19 mRNA was detected in the erythema nodosum (EN)-like lesion of BD [27].

A significant increase in IL-17- and IFN-γ-expressing CD4+ memory T cells was observed in patients with active BD compared with control groups [28]. Similarly, the levels of IL-17, IL-23, IL-12/IL-23p40, and IFN-γ in serum and supernatants were increased in active BD patients compared with control groups [28]. IFN-γ-secreting Th17 cells were elevated in BD patients [27–29]. Touzot M et al. reported that IL-17 was not inhibited by IFN-α in BD and IFN-α increased IFN-γ level in memory CD4+ T cells in BD [31]. Thus, BD is associated with a mixture of TH1/Th17 cytokine.

Patients with BD in remission expressed low Th17 levels compared to active BD [21, 24, 28]. Thus, the population of Th17 cells is correlated with BD activity [16, 22].

More recently, Lucherini et al. [32] reported that serum amyloid A (SAA) induced Th17 polarization rather than Th1 differentiation from CD4+ T cells in BD patients. A critical regulation of Th17 may be the functional link between acute SAA increase and the induction of Th17-mediated inflammatory response in BD.

Deniz et al. [33] reported that under Th17-stimulating conditions, T cells express both IL-17 and IFN-γ in BD. In addition, they speculated that more prominent IL-17 and IFN-γ production by all lymphocyte subsets in BD may be associated with the increased innate responses, early tissue neutrophil infiltrations, and late adaptive immunity in BD.

3.3 IL-23-IL-17 axis

Recently, it is reported that IL-23R is principal for the differentiation of IL-17-producing effector T cells in vivo [34]. IL-23 was essential to preserve and to generate Th17 cells even in the absence of TGF-β [35]. The IL-23-IL-17 axis is crucial for the inflammation in BD [23]. Elevated levels of IL-23 and IL-17 [21, 28] were seen in peripheral blood mononuclear cells (PBMC) from active BD patients [23]. Recombinant IL-23 stimulated IL-17 in CD4+ T cells in BD patients [15, 23]. Recently, IL-23R, IL-12RB2, and IL-10 were identified as BD susceptibility loci by genetic surveys including GWAS [3, 4]. It is reported that the genetic variation of IL-17F and IL-23 A is associated with BD [36]. Jiang et al. [37] reported that IL-23R gene polymorphism enhanced the expression of the IL-23 R and IL-17 in BD patients.

3.4 The suppressive effect of IL-27 on Th17 cell differentiation

IL-27 is a regulator of the proinflammatory T cell response. In mouse, IL-27 plays a negative role in Th17 cell differentiation. It is reported that decreased level of IL-27 in patients with active BD [38] and decreased IL-27 expression was correlated with uveitis activity in patients with BD [38]. IL-27 inhibited human Th17 cell differentiation by upregulation of the expression of interferon regulatory factor (IRF) 8 [38]. Previous studies have shown that the presence of IL-27 limits Th17-mediated uveitis [39].

4. IL-21 and IL-26 in BD

It was reported that the expression of IL-21 was elevated in the serum of active BD patiens, and that this promoted Th17 differentiation [16]. IL-26 levels in cerebrospinal fluid and bronchoalveolar lavage fluid in BD patients showed positive correlations with IL-17 level. IL-26-stimulated $CD4^{+}$ T cells and monocytes promote the generation of Th17 and suppress regulatory T cell cytokines [40].

5. Uveitis in BD

Some investigators reported that IL-17 [15, 41], IL-23, and IFN-γ in the sera and aqueous humor significantly increased in BD patients with active uveitis compared with BD patients without active uveitis and HC [23]. It is also reported that IFN-γ-producing and IL-17-producing T cells in BD patients with active uveitis were increased [15, 23, 38]. Thus, the IL-23/IL-17 pathway plays an important role in active uveitis in BD patients. Activated CD4+ T cells obtained from BD patients produce TNF-α in vitro. Chi et al. demonstrated that IL-12 exerted its inhibitory effect on IL-17 through IFN-γ. They also reported that recombinant-IL-23 (rIL-23) can promote the production of IL-17 by CD4+ T cells in BD patients [23]. Jiang et al. reported an association of rs17375018 in the IL-23R gene with uveitis in BD patients [41]. Taken together, elevated levels of IL-17 may be associated with the intraocular inflammation of BD patients [15, 23].

6. Oral and genital ulcer and articular symptoms

Alpsoy et al. reported that IL-17 levels of BD patients with active stages of oral and genial ulcers and articular symptoms were higher than BD patients with inactive stages of these symptoms [42]. They also found that the percentage of CD4+ IL-17+, IL-17, and CD4− IL-17+ T cells was significantly elevated after *E. coli* and PHA stimulation in active organ involvement.

7. Skin

Hamzaoui et al. confirmed that the presence of an important population of IL-17+ cells infiltrates the erythema nodosum-like eruption in BD skin lesions using antibodies to IL-17A [21]. Shimizu et al. demonstrated that IFN-γ + IL-17 + -producing cells were dominant, and some of them were CD4+ cells in BD-EN compared with healthy controls [30]. Th17 cells are elevated in circulation and distribution over the skin lesions of BD patient. Ekinci et al. reported that serum IL-17A levels were markedly elevated in BD patients with active stages of oral ulcers or genital ulcers compared with inactive stage of these symptoms [22]. They also studied the proportion of IL-17-secreting cells in patients with active organ involvement, showing that the percentage of IL-17, CD4− IL-17+ cells, and CD4+ IL-17+ cells was significantly elevated [20, 22]. This finding indicated that Th17 and IL-17 pathway has a crucial role in the acute attack of the disease.

8. Entero-BD

Gastrointestinal involvement is an important complication of BD. Emmi et al. [43] found that T cells at the intestinal mucosal level produce a high amount of TNF-α and in the early stage of BD. Both Th17 and Th1 cells drive inflammation and mucosal damage though long-lasting cytokine production [44]. Imamura et al. reported the infiltration of CD4+ and CD8+ T cells in the intestine of BD patient, like the expression of mRNAs of proinflammatory and Th1 cytokines/chemokines [45]. Recently, IL-17A, IL-23R, and STAT4 polymorphisms may be involved in the pathogenesis of intestinal involvement in Korean BD patients [46]. On the other hand, Ferrante et al. reported that the serum and mRNA level of IL-23 and IL-17 in entero-BD were not different from those with control groups; thus a Th1 but not a Th17 response occurs with entero-BD [47]. More studies are needed to reveal the role of IL-17 in intestinal involvement of BD.

9. Neuro-BD

The expression of RAR-related orphan receptor C (RORC), which is the master transcription factor of Th17 cells, was elevated in the cerebrospinal fluid (CSF) of patients with neuro-BD [48]. In the CSF, the Th17/regulatory T cell (Treg) ratio was elevated [49]. It was reported that increased level of IL-17 secretion in the sera of BD patients and the elevated expression of transcription factors for Th17 cells were shown in the CSF were detected with neuro-BD patients [48]. It is reported that IL-17A- and IL-21-producing T cells in the CSF, brain parenchyma inflammatory infiltrates, and intra-cerebral blood vessels from patients with active BD and neuro-BD [16]. The stimulation of CD4+ T cells with IL-21 increased Th1 and Th17 differentiation and decreased the regulatory T cells [16]. Conversely, IL-21 blockade with an IL21R-Fc restored the Th17 and regulatory T cell homeostasis in BD patients [16]. On the other hand, Saruhan-Direskeneli et al. [49] reported that, both in serum and the CSF, IL-17 was not detectable in BD patients with CNS involvement. Thus, the pathogenesis of IL-17 in neuro-BD remains controversial.

10. Polymorphisms

The signaling molecules and Th1- and Th17-related cytokines are involved in the pathogenesis of BD [50–52]. Several reports showed that polymorphisms of Th17-related cytokines and receptors, such as IL-17F, IL-23R, and IL-23 A, were related to BD susceptibility in Korean and Chinese [41, 53, 54]. STAT4 is necessary for the increase of Th17 cells activated by IL-23. Functional studies showed that the risk SNPs in the STAT4 gene took part in BD might affect the expression of STAT4 and production of IL-17 [55]. The haplotype of IL-17A had a relation to the entero-BD risk, where those of IL-23R are protected against disease expansion. The interactions of IL-23R, IL-17A, and STAT4 SNPs modify the susceptibility to intestinal BD, suggesting the crucial role of the IL-17/IL-23 axis in the pathogenesis of intestinal BD [56].

11. Plasticity

Recently, plasticity of Th17 and Th17 cells means that they can produce Th1 (IFN-γ)- or Th2 (IL-4)-type cytokines under inflammation [57, 58]. Th17 cells are able to change IFN-γ-expressing T cells in mouse Th1 disease models, which are named Th17/Th1 cells, IFN-γ-expressing Th17 cells, or Th1-like cells. The expression of RORC is not fixed in T cells, and the plasticity of Th17 cells was recognized in murine models in vivo [45]; this conception was applied to human diseases [59, 60]. Geri et al. demonstrated that the frequencies of IFN-γ CD4+ T cells and IL-17+ CD4+ T cells were increased in the CSF than in PBMC in BD patients [16]. Th1 and Th17 cells may be complicated at different steps in inflammatory process, and more Th17 cells were generated than Th1 cells during the inflammatory process. The elevated level in Th17/Treg cells and Th17/Th1 ratios is correlated with the expanse of inflammation. In BD, plasticity exists between Th1, Th17, and Treg cells during inflammation at inflammatory sites and in the peripheral circulation [61]. The low levels of Th17 in remission BD compared with active BD may be due to a conversion of Th17 cells into Treg cells. The differentiation of Treg cells into Th17 cells was involved in the downregulation of FoxP3 expression and the suppressor function. Foxp3 inhibits Th17 differentiation by antagonizing the RORγt function [62]. Sonmez et al. [63] reported that IL-17A/F levels increased parallel to IL-23 levels in BD and IL-35 levels were lower in active BD patients than the inactive BD patients, which may be a plasticity between Th17 and Treg cells according to the state of disease activity.

12. Therapy

12.1 Cyclosporine A (CsA)

CsA is effective for reducing the severity of intraocular inflammation of BD. Chi et al. reported that CsA has an effect on both IFN-γ and IL-17 productions in vitro and in vivo. In vitro, it was shown that CsA inhibited IL-17 production from PBMC of BD patients. In vivo, the improvement of intraocular inflammation in BD was accompanied by the suppression of both IFN-γ and IL-17 productions after CsA administration [24]. Therefore, it is suggested that the efficacy of CsA on uveitis in BD is through the inhibition of IFN-γ and IL-17 production.

12.2 Antibodies to IFN-α

Type I IFNs were able to inhibit IL-17 production by PBMC. Recombinant IFN-α has been used to treat BD [57]. Liu et al. reported that significantly higher levels of IL-17 are detected in active BD patients and stimulation with IFN-α decrease IL-17 production [17]. In vitro study showed that IFN-α does not directly regulate the Th1/Th17 balance in BD but rather promotes a regulatory Th1 response through IL-10 secretion [63]. IFN-α activity was mediated via STAT2 phosphorylation [17]. IFN-α upregulates the gene expression of IL-27, a negative regulator of Th17 cells [64].

12.3 Anti-TNF-α therapy

TNF-α has been detected in patients with BD [5]. Anti-TNF-α blockade can increase Tregs [46] and prevent effector T cell differentiation in BD patients with uveitis [14, 65, 66]. It was demonstrated that the production of IL-17 by polarized Th17 cell lines exposed to infliximab in vitro or fresh CD4+ T cells from BD patients being treated with infliximab was decreased and the RORγt in T cells was also decreased. Therefore, TNF-α is needed for Th17 differentiation in BD. CD4+ T cells exposed to anti-TNF-α blockade may transform into Treg cells. Anti-TNF-α therapy-induced Treg cells from BD patients restrained the activation of target T cells [14]. Anti-TNF-α agents have efficacy for uveitis, neurological and gastrointestinal involvement, and vessel diseases in BD [66]. Taken together, the Th17/Treg cell balance may be crucial for the inflammation in BD [45, 58].

12.4 Antibodies to IL-17A

IL-17A has a crucial role in deterioration of eye disease and oral ulcers, genital ulcers, and articular symptoms [21–23]. IL-17A from active BD patients can increase the expression of adhesion molecule mRNA. Therapy with antibodies to IL-17A decreased the production of adhesion molecules [21, 67]. Some reported [68–70] that secukinumab improved active mucocutaneous manifestation refractory to previous treatment such as colchicine, conventional DMARDs, and anti-TNF-α agent [69], and refractory oral ulcers [68]. Thus, therapeutic modalities attempting to evaluate new approaches to eliminate the over activities of IL-17A and/or the IL-23/IL-17 pathway may clarify the pathological importance of Il-17A and Th17 cells in BD patients.

13. Other therapeutic strategies

It is reported that suppression of microRNA-155 reduced the amount of pathogenic IL-17-expressing T cells [71].

13.1 Prognostic biomarker

The proportion of Th17 cells was increased, which was related with the increasing levels of IL-17, IL-23, and RORγt mRNA expression in BD patients. Ahmadi et al. [72] reported that T cell-associated miRNA expression levels, miR-25, miR-106b, miR-326, and miR-93 were significantly unregulated in PBMCs in BD patients; thus the evaluation of immune cells and related miRNA profile may serve as prognostic biomarker.

14. Conclusion

BD is predominated by Th1 and Th17 immune responses. Th17 cells are associated with the active inflammation of BD. Thus, IL-23-IL-17 axis and Th1/Th17-type immune responses are crucial for inflammation and have a pathologic role in BD.

Conflict of interest

We have no conflict of interest.

Acronyms and abbreviations

BD	Behçet's disease
IL	interleukin
TNF	tumor necrosis factor
RORC	RAR-related orphan receptor C
CRP	C-reactive protein
SAA	serum amyloid A
IFN	interferon
PBMC	peripheral blood mononuclear cells
CsA	cyclosporine A
Th	T helper
Treg	regulatory T cell

Author details

Yuki Nanke[1,2]* and Shigeru Kotake[2]

1 Institute of Rheumatology, Tokyo Women's Medical University, Tokyo, Japan

2 Division of Rheumatology, First Department of Comprehensive Medicine, Jichi Medical University Saitama Medical Center, Saitama, Japan

*Address all correspondence to: ynn@twmu.ac.jp

References

[1] Nanke Y, Kotake S, Ogasawara K, Shimakawa M, Takasawa S, Ujihara H, et al. Raised plasma adrenomedullin level in Behçet's disease patients. Modern Rheumatology. 2003;**13**:139-142. DOI: 10.3109/s10165-002-0213-6

[2] Greco A, De Virgilio A, Ralli M, Ciofalo A, Mancini P, Attanasio G, et al. Behçet's disease: New insights into pathophysiology, clinical features and treatment options. Autoimmunity Reviews. 2018;**17**(6):567-575. DOI: 10.1016/j.autrev.2017.12.006

[3] Misuki N, Meguro A, Ota M, Ohno S, Shiota T, Kawagoe T, et al. Genome-wide association studies identify IL23R-IL12 RB 2 and IL10. Nature Genetics. 2010;**42**:703-706. DOI: 10.1038/ng.624

[4] Remers EF, Cosan F, Kirino Y, Ombrello MJ, Abaci N, Satorius C, et al. Genome wide association study identifies variants in the MHC class I, IL-10, and IL-23R-IL12 RB2 regions associated with Behçet's disease. Nature Genetics. 2010;**42**(8):698-702. DOI: 10.1038/ng.625

[5] Hamzaoui K, Hamzaoui A, Guemira F, Bessioud M, Ayed K. Cytokine profile in Behçet's disease patients. Relationship with disease activity. Scandinavian Journal of Rheumatology. 2002;**31**(4):205-210

[6] Ben Ahmed M, Houman H, Miled M, Dellagi K, Louzir H. Involvement of chemokines and Th1 cytokines in the pathogenesis of mucocutaneous lesions of Behçet's disease. Arthritis and Rheumatism. 2004;**50**(7):2291-2295

[7] Direskeneli H, Fujita H, Akdis CA. Regulation of TH17 and regulatory T cells in patients with Behçet's disease. The Journal of Allergy and Clinical Immunology. 2011;**128**(3):665-666. DOI: 10.1016/j.jaci.2011.07.008

[8] Yoshimura T, Sonoda KH, Miyazaki Y, Iwakura Y, Ishibashi T, Yoshimura A, et al. Differential roles for IFN-gamma and IL-17 in experimental autoimmune uveoretinitis. International Immunology. 2008;**20**(2):209-214

[9] Yoshimura T, Sonoda KH, Ohguro N, Ohsugi Y, Ishibashi T, Cua DJ, et al. Involvement of Th17 cells and the effect of anti-IL-6 therapy in autoimmune uveitis. Rheumatology (Oxford). 2009;**48**:347-354. DOI: 10.1093/rheumatology/ken489

[10] Cui Y, Shao H, Lan C, Nian H, O'Brien RL, Born WK, et al. Major role of gamma delta T cells in the generation of IL-17+ uveitogenic T cells. Journal of Immunology. 2009;**183**:560-567. DOI: 10.4049/jimmunol.0900241

[11] Oh K, Byoun OJ, Ham DI, Kim YS, Lee DS. Invariant NKT cells regulate experimental autoimmune uveitis through inhibition of Th17 differentiation. European Journal of Immunology. 2011;**41**:392-402. DOI: 10.1002/eji.201040569

[12] Choi B, Hwang Y, Kwon HJ, et al. Tumor necrosis factor alpha small interfering RNA decreases herpes simplex virus-induced inflammation in a mouse model. Journal of Dermatological Science. 2008;**52**(2):87-97. DOI: 10.1016/j.jdermsci.2008.05.001

[13] Shim J, Byun HO, Lee YD, Lee ES, Sohn S. Interleukin-6 small interfering RNA improved the herpes simplex virus-induced systemic inflammation in vivo Behçet's disease-like mouse model. Gene Therapy. 2009;**16**(3):415-425. DOI: 10.1038/gt.2008.180

[14] Sugita S, Kawazoe Y, Imai A, Yamada Y, Horie S, Mochizuki M. Inhibition of Th 17 differentiation by anti-ANF-alpha therapy in uveitis patients with Behçet's disease. Arthritis

Research & Therapy. 2012;**14**(3):R99. DOI: 10.1186/ar3824

[15] Chi W, Zhou X, Yang P, Liu X, Zhou H, Huang X, et al. Upregulated IL-23 and IL-17 in Behçet's patients with active uveitis. Investigative Ophthalmology & Visual Science. 2008;**49**(7):3058-3064. DOI: 10.1167/iovs.07-1390

[16] Geri G, Terrier B, Rosenzwajg M, Wechsler B, Touzot M, Seilhean D, et al. Critical role of IL-21 in modulating TH 17 and regulatory T cells in Behçet's disease. The Journal of Allergy and Clinical Immunology. 2011;**128**(3):655-664. DOI: 10.1016/j.jaci.2011.05.029

[17] Liu X, Yang P, Wang C, Li F, Kijlstra A. IFN-α blocks IL-17 production by peripheral blood mononuclear cells in Behçet's disease. Rheumatology. 2011;**50**(2):293-298. DOI: 10.1093/rheumatology/keq330

[18] Yasuoka H, Chen Z, Takeuchi T, Kuwana M. Th 17 is involved in the pathogenesis of Behçet's disease via CCl20-CCR6 axis. Arthritis Research & Therapy. 2012;**14**:79

[19] Al-Zifzaf DS, Mokbel AN, Abdelaziz DM. Interleukin-17 in Behçet's disease. Relation with clinical picture and disease activity. Egyptian Rheumatology & Rehabiliation. 2015;**42**:34-38

[20] Alpsoy E. Behçet's disease: A comprehensive review with a focus on epidemiology, etiology and clinical features, and management of mucocutaneous lesions. The Journal of Dermatology. 2016;**43**(6):620-632. DOI: 10.1111/1346-8138.13381

[21] Hamzaoui K, Bouali E, Ghorbel I, Khanfir M, Houman H, Hamzaoui A. Expression of Th17 and RORγt mRNA in Behçet's disease. Medical Science Monitor. 2011;**17**:CR227-CR234

[22] Ekinci NS, Alpsoy E, karakas AA, et al. IL-17A has an important role in the acute attacks of Behçet's disease. The Journal of Investigative Dermatology. 2010;**130**(8):2136-2138. DOI: 10.1038/jid.2010.114

[23] Chi W, Zhou X, Yang P, Chen L. CD4+ T cells from Behçet patients produced high levels of IL-17. Eye Science. 2011;**26**:65-69. DOI: 10.3969/j.issn.1000-4432.2011.02.013

[24] Chi W, Yang P, Zhu X, et al. Production of interleukin-17 in Behçet's disease is inhibited by cyclosporine A. Molecular Vision. 2010;**16**:880-886

[25] Cetin EA, Cosan F, Cefle A, Deniz G. IL-22-secreting Th22 and IFN-γ-secreting Th17 cells in Behçet's disease. Modern Rheumatology. 2014;**24**(5):802-807. DOI: 10.3109/14397595.2013.879414

[26] Kim J, Park JA, Lee EY, Lee YJ, Song YW, Lee EB. Imbalance of Th17 to Th1 cells in Behçet's disease. Clinical and Experimental Rheumatology. 2010;**60**:S16-S19

[27] Lew W, Chang JY, Jung JY, Bang D. Increased expression of interleukin-23 p19 mRNA in erythema nodosum-like of Behçet's disease. The British Journal of Dermatology. 2008;**158**(3):505-511. DOI: 10.1111/j.1365-2133.2007.08403.x

[28] Na SY, Park MJ, Park S, Lee ES. Up-regulation of Th 17 and related cytokines in Behçet's disease corresponding to disease activity. Clinical and Experimental Rheumatology. 2013;**77**:32-40

[29] Aktas Cetin E, Cosan F, Cefle A, Deniz G. IL-22-secreting Th22 and IFN-γ in patients with Behçet's disease. Modern Rheumatology. 2014;**24**(5):802-807. DOI: 10.3109/14397595.2013.879414

[30] Shimizu J, Takai K, Fujiwara N, Arimitsu N, Ueda Y, Wakisaka S, et al. Excessive CD4+ T cells

co-expessing interleukin-17 and interferon-α in patients with Behçet's disease. Clinical and Experimental Immunology. 2012;**168**(1):68-74. DOI: 10.1111/j.1365-2249.2011.04543.x

[31] Touzot M, Cacoub P, Bodaghi B, Soumelis V, Saadoun D. INF-α induces IL-10 production and tilt the balance between Th1 and Th17 in Behçet's diseases. Autoimmunity Reviews. 2015;**14**(5):370-375. DOI: 10.1016/j.autrev.2014.12.009

[32] Lucherini OM, Lopalco G, Cantnrini L, Emmi R, Lopalco A, Venerito V, et al. Critical regulation of Th17 cell differentiation by serum amyloid-A signaling in Behçet's disease. Immunology Letters. 2018;**201**:38-44. DOI: 10.1016/j.imlet.2018.10.013

[33] Deniz R, Tulunay-Virlan A, TureOzdemir F, Unal AU, Ozen G, Alibaz-Oner F, et al. Th 17-inducing conditions lead to in vitro activation of both Th17 and Th1 responses in Behçet's disease. Immunological Investigations. 2017;**46**(5):518-525. DOI: 10.1080/08820139.2017.1306865

[34] McGeachy MJ, Chen Y, Tato CM, et al. The interleukin-23 receptor is essential for the terminal differentiation of interleukin 17-producing effector T helper cells in vivo. Nature Immunology. 2009;**10**(3):314-324. DOI: 10.1038/ni.1698

[35] Das J, Ren G, Zhang L, et al. Transforming growth factor beta is dispensable for the molecular orchestration of Th17 cell differentiation. The Journal of Experimental Medicine. 2009;**206**(11):2407-2416. DOI: 10.1084/jem.20082286

[36] Hou S, Liao D, Zhang J, Fang J, Chen L, Qi J, et al. Genetic variation of IL17F and Il23A show associations with Behçet's disease and Vogt-Koyanagi-Harada syndrome. American Journal of Ophthalmology. 2015;**122**(3):518-523. DOI: 10.1016/j.ophtha.2014.09.025

[37] Jiang Z, Henein L, Tao Y, Tao L. Interleukin-23 receptor gene polymorphism may enhance expression of the IL-23 receptor, Il-17, TNF-α and Il-6 in Behçet's disease. PLoS ONE. 2015;**10**(7):e0134632. DOI: 10.1371/journal.pone.0134632

[38] Wang C, Tian Y, Ye Z, Kijlstra A, Zhou Y, Yang P. Decreased interleukin 27 expression is associated with active uveitis in Behçet's disease. Arthritis Research & Therapy. 2014;**16**(3):R117. DOI: 10.1186/ar4570

[39] Amadi-Obi A, Yu CR, Liu X, Mahdi RM, Clarke GL, Nussenball RB, et al. Th17 cells contribute to uveitis and scleritis and are expanded by IL-2 and inhibited by IL-27/STAT1. Nature Medicine. 2007;**13**(6):711-718

[40] Kaabachi W, Bouali E, Berraies A, Dhifallh IB, Hamzaoui K, Hamzaoui A. Interleukin-26 is overexpressed in Behçet's disease and enhances Th17 related-cytokines. Immunology Letters. 2017;**190**:177-184. DOI: 10.1016/j.imlet.2017.08.008

[41] Jiang Z, Yang P, Hou S, Du L, Xie L, Zhou H, et al. IL-23R gene confers susceptibility to Behçet's disease in a Chinese Han population. Annals of the Rheumatic Diseases. 2010;**69**(7):1325-1328. DOI: 10.1136/ard.2009.119420

[42] Alpsoy E. Behçet's disease: A comprehensive review with a focus on epidemiology, etiology and clinical features, and management of mucocutaneous lesions. The Journal of Dermatology. 2016;**43**:620-632

[43] Emmi G, Silvestri E, Bella CD, Grassi A, Benagiano M, Cianchi F,

et al. Cytotoxic Th1 and Th17 cells infiltrate the intestinal mucosa of Behest patients and exhibit high levels of TNF-α in early phases of the disease. Medicine (Baltimore). 2016;**95**(49):e5516

[44] Emmi G, Silvestri E, Bella CD, Grassi A, Benagiano M, Cianchi F, et al. Cytotoxic Th1 and Th17 cells infiltrate the intestinal mucosa of Behçet patients and exhibit high levels of TNF-α in early phases of the disease. Medicine (Baltimore). 2016;**95**(49):e5516

[45] Imamura Y, Kurokawa MS, Yoshikawa H, et al. Involvement of Th1 cells and heat shock protein 60 in the pathogenesis of interstinal Behçet's disease. Clinical & Experimental Immunology. 2005;**139**(2):371-378

[46] Sugita S, Yamada Y, Kaneko S, et al. Induction of regulatory T cells by infliximab in Behçet's disease. Investigative Ophthalmology & Visual Science. 2011;**52**:476-484

[47] Ferrante A, Ciccia F, Principato A, Giardina AR, Impastato R, Peralta S, et al. A Th1 but not a Th17 response in present in the gastrointestinal involvement of Behçet's disease. Clinical and Experimental Rheumatology. 2010;**60**:S27-S30

[48] Hamzaoui K, Borhani haghighia A, Ghorbel LB, Houman H. RORC and Foxp3 axis in cerebrospinal fluid of patients with neuro-Behçet's disease. Journal of Neuroimmunology. 2011;**233**(1-2):249-253. DOI: 10.1016/j.jneuroim.2011.01.012

[49] Saruhan-Direskeneli G, Yentur SP, Akman-Demir G, Isik N, Serdaroglu P. Cytokines and chemokines in neuro-Behçet's disease compared to multiple sclerosis and other neurological disease. Journal of Neuroimmunology. 2003;**143**:127-134

[50] Shimizu J, Izumi T, Arimitsu N, et al. Skewed TGFβ/smad signaling pathway in T cells in patients with Behçet's disease. Clinical and Experimental Rheumatology. 2012;**30**(suppl.72):S35-S39

[51] Shaharam F, Nikoopour E, Rezaei N, et al. Association of interleukin-2, interleukin-4 and transforming growth factor-beta gene polymorphisms with Behçet's disease. Clinical and Experimental Rheumatology. 2011;**30**(supple 67):S28-S31

[52] Zhang YJ, Xu WD, Duan ZH, Liu SS, Pan HF, Ye DQ. Lack of association between CTLA 4+49A/G and −318 C/T polymorphisms and Behçet's disease risk: A meta-analysis. Clinical and Experimental Rheumatology. 2012;**30**(supple 72):S46-S50

[53] Jang WC, Nam YF, Ahn YC, Lee SH, Park SH, Choe JY, et al. Interleukin-17F gene polymorphisms in Korean patients with Behçet's disease. Rheumatology International. 2008;**29**(2):173-178. DOI: 10.1007/s00296-008-0664-y

[54] Hou S, Liao D, Zhang J, Fang J, Chen L, Qi J, et al. Genetic variations of Il-17F and IL-23A show associations with Behçet's disease and Vogt-Koyanagi-Harada syndrome. Oppthalmology. 2015;**122**(3):518-523. DOI: 10.1016/j.ophtha.2014.09.025

[55] Hou S, Yang Z, Du L, Jiang Z, Shu Q, Yuanyuan C, et al. Identification of a susceptibility locus in STAT4 for Behçet's disease in Han Chinese in a genome-wide association study. Arthritis and Rheumatism. 2012;**64**(12):4104-4113. DOI: 10.1002/art.37708

[56] Kim ES, Kim SW, Moon CM, Park JJ, Kim TL, Kim WH, et al. Interactions between IL-17A, Il23R, and STAT4 polymorphisms confer susceptibility to intestinal Behçet's disease in

Korean population. Life Sciences. 2012;**90**(19-20):740-746. DOI: 10.1016/j.lfs.2012.03.017

[57] Deuter CM, Zierhat M, Mohle A, Vonthein R, Stobiger N, Kotter I. Long-term remission after cessation of interferon-a treatment in patients with severe uveitis due to Behçet's disease. Arthritis and Rheumatism. 2010;**62**(9):2796-2805. DOI: 10.1002/art.27581

[58] Harrington LE, Hatton RD, Mangan PR, Turner H, Murphy TL, Murphy KM, et al. Interleukin 17-producing CD4+ effector T cells develop via a lineage distinct from the T helper type 1 and 2 lineages. Nature Immunology. 2005;**6**(11):1123-1132

[59] Nistala K, Adams S, Cambrook H, et al. Th17 plasticity in human autoimmune arthritis is driven by the inflammatory environment. Proceedings of the National Academy of Sciences of the United States of America. 2010;**107**(33):1451-1456. DOI: 10.1073/pnas.1003852107

[60] Cosmi L, Cimaz R, Maggi L, et al. Evidence of the transient nature of the Th17 phenotype of CD4+ CD161+ T cells in the synovial fluid of patients with juvenile idiopathic arthritis. Arthritis and Rheumatism. 2011;**63**(8):2504-2515. DOI: 10.1002/art.30332

[61] Hamzaoui K. Th17 cells in Behçet's disease: A new immunoregulatory axis. Clinical and Experimental Rheumatology. 2011;**67**:S71-S76

[62] Zhou L, Lopes JE, Mark MW, et al. TGF-beta induced Foxp3 inhibits T(H)17 cell differentiation by antagonizing RORgammat function. Nature. 2008;**453**(7192):236-240. DOI: 10.1038/nature06878

[63] Sonmez C, Yucel AA, Yesil TH, et al. Correlation between IL-17A/F IL-23, IL-35 and IL-12?-23 (p40) levels in peripheral blood lymphocyte cultures and disease activity in Behçet's disease. Clinical Rheumatology. 2018;**37**(10):2797-2804

[64] Pirhonen J, Siren J, Julkunen I, Matikainen S. IFN-alpha regulates Toll-like receptor-mediated IL-27 gene expression in human macrophages. Journal of Leukocyte Biology. 2007;**82**(5):1185-1192

[65] Ohno S, Nakamura S, Hori S, Shimakawa M, Kawashima H, Mochizuki M, et al. Efficacy, safety, and pharmacokinetics of multiple administration of infliximab in Behçet's disease with refractory uveoretinitis. The Journal of Rheumatology. 2004;**31**(7):1362-1368

[66] Desbois AC, Vallet H, Domont F, Comarmond C, Cacoub P, Saadoun D. Management of severe complications in Behçet's disease with TNF inhibitors. Expert Opinion on Biological Therapy. 2017;**17**(7):853-859. DOI: 10.1080/14712598.2017.1328496

[67] Zhang R, Qian J, Guo J, Yuan YF, Xue K. Suppression of experimental autoimmune uveoretinitis by anti-IL-17 antibody. Current Eye Research. 2009;**34**(4):297-303. DOI: 10.1080/02713680902741696

[68] Mirouse A, Barete S, Monfort JB, Resche-Rigon M, Bouyer AS, Seme D, et al. Ustekinumab for Behçet's disease. Journal of Autoimmunity. 2017;**82**:41-46. DOI: 10.1016/j.jaut.2017.05.002

[69] Di Scala G, Betttiol A, Cojan RD, Finocchi M, Sillvestri E, Emmi G. Efficacy of the anti-IL-17 secukinumab in refractory Behçet's syndrome: A preliminary study. Journal of Autoimmunity. 2019;**97**:108-113. DOI: 10.1016/j.jaut.2018.09.002

[70] Baerveladt EM, Kappen JH, Thio HB, van Laar JA, van Hagen

PM, Prens EP. Successful long-term triple disease control by ustekinumab in patients with Behçet's disease, psoriasis and hidradenitis suppurativa. Annals of the Rheumatic Diseases. 2013;**72**(4):626-627. DOI: 10.1136/annrheumdis-2012-202392

[71] Na SY, Park MJ, Park S, Lee ES. MicroRNA-155 regulates the Th17 immune response by targeting Ets-1 in Behçet's disease. Clinical and Experimental Rheumatology. 2016;**34**(6):S56-S63

[72] Ahmadi M, Yousefi M, Abbaspour-Aghdam S, Dolati S, Aghebati-Maleki L, Eghbal-Fard S, et al. Disturbed Th17Treg balance, cytokines, and miRNAs in peripheral blood of patients with Behçet's disease. Journal of Cellular Physiology. 2019;**234**(4):3985-3994

Section 3

Pregnancy and Behçet's Disease

Chapter 5

Behçet's Disease and Pregnancy

Gökçe Işıl Kurmuş and Erol Koç

Abstract

Behçet's disease (BD) is a rare, chronic, multisystemic, vasculitic disease of unknown etiology. BD is characterized by recurrent oral and genital ulcers and ocular inflammation. This systemic vasculitis may also involve the joints, skin, vascular, gastrointestinal, urogenital, and central nervous system and is associated with hypercoagulability. Disease onset is commonly around the third decade of life and has a higher prevalence along the ancient "silk route." Because the disease is often diagnosed in women of childbearing age, disease activity during pregnancy and any adverse effect on obstetric and neonatal outcomes deserve special attention. Previous retrospective studies have demonstrated that BD activity usually regresses in pregnancy because of the immunomodulatory effects of both estrogen and progesterone. Furthermore, previous reports from different countries indicate that the disease course of BD during pregnancy may vary from patient to patient and even during different pregnancies in the same woman. In this chapter, we emphasize the course of the BD and pregnancy outcomes.

Keywords: Behçet's disease, pregnancy, vasculitis, clinical course, colchicine

1. Introduction

Behçet's disease (BD) is a rare, chronic, relapsing, multisystemic, and inflammatory disorder involving the oral and genital mucosa, eyes, joints, gastrointestinal, urogenital, vascular, and central nervous system [1–3]. It commonly occurs between the ages of 18 and 40, mainly affects young men, and tends to affect individuals with "silk road" bloodlines (corresponding the ancient route between the Mediterranean, the Middle East, and the Far East) [2–5]. Although the etiopathogenesis of the disease still remains unknown, it has been hypothesized as a genetic predisposition determined by the human leucocyte antigen-B51 (HLA-B51) allele. Infectious agents such as herpes simplex virus 1 or *Streptococcus* species may play a role as pathogenic triggers in genetically predisposed individuals [4–12]. BD is characterized by histopathologic vasculitic changes and thrombogenicity, which are common to all involved organs. Vessels of all sizes are affected, both in the arterial and venous systems, with venous involvement being more common than arterial involvement [1, 4].

Most BD patients at disease onset are in their reproductive ages. Since about half of the patients with this disease are women, BD activity during pregnancy, and obstetric and neonatal outcomes must be carefully researched. Any possible interaction between this two multisystemic condition deserves special attention [1, 13, 14]. Very little is known about the influence of BD and pregnancy to date. In few anecdotal case reports and retrospective small sample studies, both remissions and flares during pregnancy have been reported, and the effect of the disease on pregnancy remained unclear [1–4, 13–22]. Based on previous studies, it can be concluded that disease activity usually regresses during pregnancy.

2. Discussion

The variability in the activity of BD in different pregnancies may be associated with various immunomodulatory effects of estrogen and progesterone, which are significantly elevated during pregnancy. Pregnancy has been associated with suppression of humoral and cellular-mediated immunological functions [23–26]. Estrogen may have anti-inflammatory actions by stimulating anti-inflammatory interleukin (IL)-10 production and counteracting the effects of IL-12, antigen-presenting capacity, and tumor necrosis factor [26–32]. Progesterone may induce the inhibition of T cell, macrophage, and natural killer cell activity during pregnancy [24, 28–31]. Progesterone can enhance both Th2 cell polarization and Treg cell production [24–30]. Oh et al. reported the case of a young woman who experienced flares of BD during every premenstrual period [33]. This condition dramatically improved when the patient received oral contraceptive therapy. As a result, it is suggested that steady-state levels of estrogen and progesterone, during pregnancy or oral contraceptive treatment, may play a role in the suppression of BD exacerbations. Krause et al. reported that neutrophil functions such as chemotaxis and adherence were depressed during pregnancy, and this was associated with an improvement in autoimmune diseases [34]. It may be the reason for the reduced number of BD flares during pregnancy, because excessive neutrophil activation has been involved in BD pathogenesis. Ferraro et al. reported an almost complete absence of autoantibodies during pregnancy in a recent study [35].

In an extensive review of the literature, both remissions and exacerbations of BD were investigated during pregnancy, and it has been reported that disease activity may differ between pregnancies in the same women [13, 15, 35–47]. The current data is limited to retrospective studies and individual case reports. Hurt et al. reported a case of severe, recurrent, oral, and genital mucosal ulcerations and iridocyclitis during the second trimester of pregnancy [46]. Madkour and Kudwah reported prolonged mucocutaneous and articular exacerbations during pregnancy and during treatment with oral contraceptive pills, in four women with BD [47]. Farrag et al. described one case of severe vaginal and cervical ulcers in the third trimester of pregnancy, treated by prednisolone [48]. Bang et al. reported on 20 pregnancies with BD, in which 12 became exacerbated [15]. The most common lesions were oral and genital ulcers in Bang's study. Similarly, in the series of Gürler and Erdi, exacerbations were observed in most of the cases [49].

In recent studies, the main symptoms during BD flares were oral ulceration and genital ulceration, followed by skin lesions and ocular inflammation; no neurological or gastrointestinal symptoms were observed during pregnancy [3, 13, 36, 38, 46–48]. The most serious manifestations of the exacerbation were vascular complications such as Budd-Chiari syndrome and deep vein thrombosis (DVT) [3, 36, 49]. Some case reports that have been reported are severe disease flares such as DVT with nephrotic syndrome, superior vena cava thrombosis, dural sinus thrombosis, or intracardiac thrombosis [16, 19, 50, 51].

Conversely, some authors reported remissions during pregnancy in BD patients. Hamza et al. studied 21 pregnancies in eight women with BD and found remissions in 12 pregnancies [38]. In this study mainly genital ulcers were seen in nine flares during the last trimester, despite systemic corticotherapy. Marsal et al. studied 25 pregnancies in 10 women and reported 23 remissions and only 2 flares [36]. Chajek and Fainaro reported a woman with persistent BD who had remissions only during her pregnancies over a 20-year follow-up [43]. Ferraro et al. and Larsson and Baum reported two similar cases with complete remissions during pregnancy with a flare after delivery [35, 45]. In a recent study, Uzun et al. reported on 44 pregnancies in 28 women and found remission rate to be 52.3%, while exacerbation rate was 27.3% [13]. In this study in nine pregnancies, there were no changes in the clinical course of BD.

In a single retrospective study by Noel et al., the authors compared the frequencies of BD exacerbations in the periods before gestation with the rate during pregnancy [3]. They observed that the annual incidence of BD flares per patient was lower during pregnancy than during the nonobstetric period. In most series there was no association between the pregnant woman's ages, the age at onset of Behçet's disease, and the course of the disease during pregnancy. Noel et al. found that the shorter duration of BD prior to conception had the higher rate of exacerbation. In addition, they investigated that the treatment with colchicine was associated with lesser exacerbations during pregnancy. On the other hand, Seyyahi et al. considered that since BD becomes less severe with the passage of time, it is also expected to see less flares with long disease duration [52]. Moreover, patients who were treated only with colchicine had probably a milder disease, and hence, they experienced less flares during pregnancy.

In a review Ben-Chetrit reported the rate of complications ranges between 4 and 20% of pregnancies in eight different studies [14]. In these studies only Marsal et al., Jadaon et al., and Iskender et al. compared their study groups with healthy controls [1, 2, 36]. Marsal et al. reported no significant differences in the incidence of maternal and fetal complications (abortions, congenital abnormalities, perinatal death, etc.) between BD patients and healthy controls [36]. In the series of Iskender et al., the frequencies of stillbirth, preeclampsia, preterm delivery, and cesarean deliveries did not differ between groups [1]. Jadaon et al. reported the highest rate of complications (20%) of these studies and significantly more than control groups [2]. The authors considered that especially the higher rate of miscarriage, but also the elevated pregnancy complication rate, may be explained by the vasculitic process underlying the pathogenesis of BD, as well as by hypercoagulability during pregnancy in BD patients. There was no difference of the neonatal outcomes such as intrauterine growth restriction, congenital abnormalities, neonatal weight, APGAR score at 1 and 5 min, respiratory distress syndrome, intraventricular hemorrhage, convulsions, prematurity, and perinatal death between the study and control groups [2]. In the reports by Noel et al. and Nadzi et al., the rate of complications was similar (16–19%) among their BD pregnant patients [3, 53]. In these studies, the high rate of miscarriages and the high number of deliveries by cesarean section were reported. Noel et al. observed a significant association between a history of DVT in BD and the risk of obstetric complications (miscarriages and cesarean deliveries) [3]. They found that the previous venous involvement due to BD increased obstetric complications, as previously suggested by Jadaon et al. [2]. All of such patients in their cohort had experienced prior DVT, and two had associated cerebral venous thrombosis. The main obstetric complications were miscarriages for these patients. The authors considered that there was a link between venous thrombosis and the risk of default in trophoblast implantation [3]. They suggested that the antiphospholipid syndrome must be ruled out. The risk of fetal loss in BD is, however, lower than the risk in antiphospholipid syndrome [54]. Jadaon et al. thought that the presence of anti-endothelial cell antibodies in the sera of patients with BD and impaired function of vascular endothelial cells may explain the high rate of miscarriages and pregnancy complications in BD patients [2, 55, 56]. However, these observations were not reported by other retrospective studies. In addition, the outcome of pregnancies varied even during different pregnancies in the same BD patient, suggesting that it is not invariably related to BD.

Jadaon et al. observed the rate of BD patients in which patients who went into remission was significantly higher than the number of patients who had exacerbations in the postpartum period [2]. In this case control study, it was shown that patients, who went into remission or exacerbation during pregnancy, tend to continue in the same direction after delivery. When the rate of remissions and exacerbations during pregnancy and postpartum period was compared, they found that the difference between the rate of remissions and exacerbations during pregnancy and postpartum for each of the women was not significant. They reported that there was no difference in disease activity during pregnancy and postpartum between HLAB51-positive and HLAB51-negative BD patients. In this study the number of pregnancies that were conceived under treatment was as follows: 29 of 77 patients with corticosteroids, 1 with colchicine, 1 with insulin, and 5 with heparin [2]. Hamza et al. reported exacerbations of BD in nine pregnancies despite corticosteroid treatment (10–15 mg/day) but no significant obstetric complications [38]. In a 20 case series reported by Marsal et al., 3 patients with corticosteroids, 1 patient with colchicine, and 1 patient with cyclosporine all discontinued the treatments at the onset of the pregnancy, due to concerns regarding adverse effects [36].

Many of the medications used in the treatment of BD are safe to use during pregnancy. These include corticosteroids, cyclosporine, and azathioprine. There is now growing evidence to suggest that colchicine is also safe to use in pregnancy, and previous concerns about associations with fetal chromosomal abnormalities have not been proven. The question of whether colchicine treatment is safe during pregnancy is important, because colchicine crosses the human placenta [3]. Despite the antimitotic effects of colchicine, the safety of this drug during pregnancy was recently assessed in a prospective comparative cohort study in which 238 colchicine-exposed pregnancies were followed up [57]. Increase in teratogenicity or congenital abnormalities was not observed. This finding is consistent with previous reports and underlines the safety of colchicine during pregnancy [58]. There is no agreement on the therapy of deep venous thrombosis and PE in BD [16]. Systemic anticoagulation with conventional agents including aspirin and low-molecular-weight heparin (LMWH) is usually applied because of hypercoagulability of pregnancy, but lack of response or recurrence may occur if immunosuppressive therapy is not continued [59].

New agents such as the anti-TNF-alpha monoclonal antibodies such as infliximab and etanercept have been used to treat inflammatory conditions in pregnancy and appear safe. There is no report that exposure to TNF inhibitors is toxic to the developing fetus. However, due to the limitations of available data and lack of controlled trials, there is not sufficient evidence to demonstrate the safety of the fetus exposed to TNF inhibitors during pregnancy. Moreover, the long-term safety of the infant is uncertain. If possible, discontinuation of the TNF inhibitor is desirable during pregnancy. If it appears to be necessary to use a TNF inhibitor to control the disease activity during mid and late pregnancy, then inoculations of live vaccine after birth pose a problem [20, 60]. It was reported that an infant born from a patient with Crohn's disease and exposed to infliximab during pregnancy died due to disseminated BCG because of a live vaccine received at 3 months of age [61]. Therefore, any infant exposed to anti-TNF monoclonal antibody in the uterus should be protected from the administration of a live vaccine until at least 6 months from birth or until the drug disappears from the serum [20]. Data on more than 300 pregnancies showed that infliximab carries low fetal risk during conception and the first two trimesters but suggests considering discontinuation in the early third trimester to minimize late fetal exposure to the risk of neonatal immunosuppression [62]. However, if treatment needs to be continued to keep the BD controlled, then the advantages probably outweigh the theoretical disadvantages. In a case report, a 30-year-old woman diagnosed with BD at 12 weeks of pregnancy was successfully treated with infliximab, 5 mg/kg repeated dosages after 18 weeks of pregnancy, with improvement in all symptoms and normal full-term delivery [21]. A 36-year-old Japanese woman with intestinal BD (a recurrent ileocecal ulcer) was treated with adalimumab [20]. In this case, infliximab treatment showed secondary failure, so infliximab was switched to adalimumab. After the third injection of adalimumab, the patient was unexpectedly 4-week pregnant. Adalimumab was continued until the 20 weeks of pregnancy. Remission of the disease activity during pregnancy, the disappearance of ileocecal ulcer after delivery was reported, and the birth was uneventful in this case. It was also reported that adalimumab was detected in the umbilical blood after 119 days from the last infusion. The placental transition and timing of neonatal vaccination should be considered in cases of pregnancy with TNF antibody therapy [20].

Thalidomide is an effective treatment of oral and genital ulceration in BD but should never be used in pregnancy or in the absence of effective contraception because of its teratogenicity. Mycophenolate mofetil may also cause fetal malformations and should ideally be discontinued prior to pregnancy. It may sometimes be replaced with azathioprine. Disease-modifying drugs such as low-dose methotrexate and cytotoxic drugs such as chlorambucil and cyclophosphamide used in BD to treat inflammation of the brain and eye should also be avoided when planning a pregnancy as these medications may cause fetal abnormalities. These drugs should be discontinued at least 3 months prior to conception and alternative safe medications commenced if necessary [63].

During lactation the risk of taking medication that may suppress neonatal immune system must be balanced against the many benefits that breast milk confers and the risk of disease relapsing if medication is not taken. Prednisolone and azathioprine are safe to use during lactation, and only low concentrations of cyclosporine are transferred to the breast milk, so these may be safe as well. Similarly colchicine, which is secreted into breast milk, has had no adverse side effects associated with its use in lactation [57]. Other agents such as infliximab and etanercept are not thought to be secreted in breast milk, but there are as yet no data on whether these drugs are safe to use in lactation [20, 21].

3. Conclusions

It seems that pregnancy in general does not have harmful effects on the natural course of BD at all, though the limited number of cases reported and the lack of prospective studies. When the data from all the published series were analyzed, it has been considered that more than 50% of BD patients will improve remission during pregnancy. However, the BD activity usually regresses during pregnancy, and it is more recommended that due to the diverse course of the disease among different patients with the various clinical presentations and organ involvement, the disease course will differ. In some patients, the disease will go into remission, and in others, it will exacerbate during pregnancy. The variability in BD course during pregnancy is not limited to different patients. Even in the same patient, in one pregnancy, the disease may remain stable, while in a subsequent one, the disease exacerbates. There was no association between the number of pregnancy and the natural course of the disease.

Author details

Gökçe Işıl Kurmuş[1*] and Erol Koç[2]

1 Department of Dermatology, Istinye University School of Medicine, Istanbul, Turkey

2 Department of Dermatology, Medical Park Ankara Hospital, Ankara, Turkey

*Address all correspondence to: gokce.kurmus@istinye.edu.tr

References

[1] Iskender C, Yasar O, Kaymak O, Yaman ST, Uygur D, Danisman N. Behçet's disease and pregnancy: A retrospective analysis of course of disease and pregnancy outcome. The Journal of Obstetrics and Gynaecology Research. 2014;**40**:1598-1602. DOI: 10.1111/jog.12386

[2] Jadaon J, Shushan A, Ezra Y, Sela HY, Ozcan C, Rojansky N. Behçet's disease and pregnancy. Acta Obstetricia et Gynecologica Scandinavica. 2005;**84**:939-944. DOI: 10.1111/j.0001-6349.2005.00761.x

[3] Noel N, Wechsler B, Nizard J, Costedoat-Chalumeau N, Boutin du LT, Dommergues M, et al. Behçet's disease and pregnancy. Arthritis and Rheumatism. 2013;**65**:2450-2456. DOI: 10.1002/art.38052

[4] Xu C, Bao S. Behçet's disease and pregnancy: A case report and literature review. American Journal of Reproductive Immunology. 2017;**77**. DOI: 10.1111/aji.12530

[5] Bang D. Clinical spectrum of Behçet's disease. The Journal of Dermatology. 2001;**28**:610-613. DOI: 10.1111/j.1346-8138.2001.tb00044.x

[6] Ugurlu N, Bozkurt S, Bacanli A, Akman-Karakas A, Uzun S, Alpsoy E. The natural course and factors affecting severity of Behçet's disease: A single-center cohort of 368 patients. Rheumatology International. 2015;**35**:2103-2107. DOI: 10.1007/s00296-015-3310-5

[7] Yücel A, Sönmezoğlu Marakli S, Aksungur VL, Uzun S, Sertdemir Y, Alpsoy E. Clinical evaluation of Behçet's disease: A five year follow-up study. The Journal of Dermatology. 2005;**32**:365-370. DOI: 10.1111/j.1346-8138.2005.tb00908.x

[8] Leccese P, Alpsoy E. Behçet's disease: An overview of etiopathogenesis. Frontiers in Immunology. 2019;**10**(10):1067. DOI: 10.3389/fimmu.2019.01067

[9] Alpsoy E. Behçet's disease: A comprehensive review with a focus on epidemiology, etiology and clinical features, and management of mucocutaneous lesions. The Journal of Dermatology. 2016;**43**:620-632. DOI: 10.1111/1346-8138.13381

[10] Alpsoy E, Zouboulis CC, Ehrlich GE. Mucocutaneous lesions of Behçet's disease. Yonsei Medical Journal. 2007;**31**(48):573-585. DOI: 10.3349/ymj.2007.48.4.573

[11] Alpsoy E, Donmez L, Bacanli A, Apaydin C, Butun B. Review of the chronology of clinical manifestations in 60 patients with Behçet's disease. Dermatology. 2003;**207**:354-356. DOI: 10.1159/000074113

[12] Ekinci NS, Alpsoy E, Karakas AA, Yilmaz SB, Yegin O. IL-17A has an important role in the acute attacks of Behçet's disease. The Journal of Investigative Dermatology. 2010;**130**:2136-2138. DOI: 10.1038/jid.2010.114

[13] Uzun S, Alpsoy E, Durdu M, Akman A. The clinical course of Behçet's disease in pregnancy: A retrospective analysis and review of the literature. The Journal of Dermatology. 2003;**30**:499-502. DOI: 10.1111/j.1346-8138.2003.tb00423.x

[14] Ben-Chetrit E. Behçet's syndrome and pregnancy: Course of the disease and pregnancy outcome. Clinical and Experimental Rheumatology. 2014;**32**:S93-S98

[15] Bang D, Chun YS, Haam IB, Lee ES, Lee S. The influence of pregnancy on Behçet's disease. Yonsei Medical Journal. 1997;**38**:437-443. DOI: 10.3349/ymj.1997.38.6.437

[16] Hiwarkar P, Stasi R, Sutherland G, Shannon M. Deep vein and intracardiac thrombosis during the post-partum period in Behçet's disease. International Journal of Hematology. 2010;**91**:679-686. DOI: 10.1007/s12185-010-0538-4

[17] Hwang I, Lee CK, Yoo B, Lee I. Necrotizing villitis and decidual vasculitis in the placentas of mothers with Behçet disease. Human Pathology. 2009;**4**:135-138. DOI: 10.1016/j.humpath.2008.04.021

[18] Mirfeizi Z, Memar B, PourZand H, Molseghi MH, Rezaei Shahmirzadi A, Abdolahi N. Ventricular endomyocardial fibrosis in a pregnant female with Behçet's disease. Asian Cardiovascular and Thoracic Annals. 2018;**26**:619-621. DOI: 10.1177/0218492316687177

[19] Wechsler B, Généreau T, Biousse V, Vauthier-Brouzes D, Seebacher J, Dormont D, et al. Pregnancy complicated by cerebral venous thrombosis in Behçet's disease. American Journal of Obstetrics and Gynecology. 1995;**173**:1627-1629. DOI: 10.1016/0002-9378(95)90663-0

[20] Fujikawa K, Endo Y, Mizokami A, Takahashi K, Tabuchi M, Ohba K, et al. Successful treatment with adalimumab for intestinal Behçet's disease during pregnancy. Internal Medicine. 2016;**55**:1375-1378. DOI: 10.2169/internalmedicine.55.6590

[21] Takayama K, Ishikawa S, Enoki T, Kojima T, Takeuchi M. Successful treatment with infliximab for Behçet disease during pregnancy. Ocular Immunology and Inflammation. 2013;**21**:321-323. DOI: 10.3109/09273948.2013.781655

[22] Higashi Y, Shimokawa M, Kawai K, Kanekura T. Granulocyte and monocyte adsorption apheresis for Behçet's disease in a pregnant woman. The Journal of Dermatology. 2013;**40**:1042-1044. DOI: 10.1111/1346-8138.12296

[23] McKay LI, Cidlowski JA. Molecular control of immune/inflammatory responses: Interactions between nuclear factor-κ B and steroid receptor-signaling pathways. Endocrine Reviews. 1999;**20**:435-459. DOI: 10.1210/edrv.20.4.0375

[24] Kanda N, Watanabe S. Regulatory roles of sex hormones in cutaneous biology and immunology. Journal of Dermatological Science. 2005;**38**:1-7. 16. DOI: 10.1016/j.jdermsci.2004.10.011

[25] Whitacre CC, Reingold SC, O'Loorey PA. A gender gap in autoimmunity. Science. 1999;**283**:1277-1278. 26. DOI: 10.1126/science.283.5406.1277

[26] Landers DV, Bronson RA, Pavia CS. Reproductive immunology. In: Stites DP, editor. Basic and Clinical Immunology. East Norwalk: Prentice Hall International Inc; 1991. pp. 91-120. 27

[27] Szekeres-Bartho J, Halasz M, Palkovics T. Progesterone in pregnancy; receptor-ligand interaction and signaling pathways. Journal of Reproductive Immunology. 2009;**83**: 60-64. DOI: 10.1016/j.jri.2009.06.262

[28] Naccasha N, Gervasi MT, Chaiworapongsa T, Berman S, Yoon BH, Maymon E, et al. Phenotypic and metabolic characteristics of monocytes and granulocytes in normal pregnancy and maternal infection. American Journal of Obstetrics and Gynecology. 2001;**185**:1118-1123. 38. DOI: 10.1067/mob.2001.117682

[29] Eksioglu-Demiralp E, Direskeneli H, Kibaroglu A, Yavuz S, Ergun T, Akoglu T. Neutrophil activation in Behçet's disease. Clinical and Experimental Rheumatology. 2001;**19**:19-24

[30] Itoh R, Takenaka T, Okitsu-Negishi S, Matsushima K, Mizogouchi M. Interleukin-8 in Behçet's disease. The Journal of Dermatology. 1994;**21**:397-404. DOI: 10.1111/j.1346-8138.1994.tb01762.x

[31] Sayinalp N, Özcebe OI, Özdemir O, Haznedaroglu IC, Dündar S, Kirazli S. Cytokines in Behçet's disease. The Journal of Rheumatology. 1996;**23**:321-322

[32] Alpsoy E, Cayirli C, Er H, Yilmaz E. The levels of plasma interleukin-2 and soluble interleukin-2r in Behçet's disease: A marker of disease activity. The Journal of Dermatology. 1998;**25**:513-516. DOI: 10.1111/j.1346-8138.1998.tb02446

[33] Oh SH, Kwon JY, Lee JH, Han EC, Bang D. Behçet's disease: Remission of patient symptoms after oral contraceptive therapy. Clinical and Experimental Dermatology. 2009;**34**:e88-e90. DOI: 10.1111/j.1365-2230.2008.03201.x

[34] Krause PJ, Ingardia CJ, Pontius LT. Host defense during pregnancy. Neutrophil chemotaxis and adherence. American Journal of Obstetrics and Gynecology. 1987;**157**:274-275. DOI: 10.1016/s0002-9378(87)80150-3

[35] Ferraro G, Lo Meo C, Moscarelli G, Assennato E. A case of pregnancy in a patient suffering from the Behçet syndrome: Immunological aspects. Acta Europaea Fertilitatis. 1984;**15**:67-70

[36] Marsal S, Falga C, Simeon CP, Vilardell M, Bosch JA. Behçet's disease and pregnancy relationship study. British Journal of Rheumatology. 1997;**36**:234-238

[37] Novak EM, Werneck LC, Mora AH. Behçet's syndrome with neurologic involvement. Arquivos de Neuro-Psiquiatria. 1977;**35**:146-150. 10

[38] Hamza M, Elleuch M, Zribi A. Behçet's disease and pregnancy. Annals of the Rheumatic Diseases. 1988;**47**:350. 11. DOI: 10.1136/ard.47.4.350-a

[39] Plouvier B, Devulder B. Behçet's disease. British Medical Journal. 1979;**i**:690. 12

[40] Suchenwirth RM. Behçet's disease and the nervous system—A 10 year follow-up with pregnancy. Fortschritte der Neurologie-Psychiatrie. 1984;**52**: 41-47. 14. DOI: 10.1055/s-2007-1002000

[41] Casanova JM, Gonzalez J, Munoz M, Bravo JM, Ramos J. Behçet's disease and pregnancy. Medicina Cutánea Ibero-Latino-Americana. 1987;**15**:387-391. 16

[42] Berman L, Trappler B, Jenkins T. Behçet's syndrome: A family study and the elucidation of genetic role. Annals of the Rheumatic Diseases. 1979;**38**: 118-121. 17. DOI: 10.1136/ard.38.2.118

[43] Chajek T, Fainaru M. Behçet's disease. Report of 41 cases and a review of the literature. Medicine (Baltimore). 1975;**54**:179-196. 18. DOI: 10.1097/00005792-197505000-00001

[44] Fam AG, Siminovitch KA, Carette S, From L. Neonatal Behçet's syndrome in an infant of a mother with the disease. Annals of the Rheumatic Diseases. 1981;**40**:509-512. 19. DOI: 10.1136/ard.40.5.509

[45] Larsson LG, Baum J. Behçet's syndrome in pregnancy and after the delivery. The Journal of Rheumatology. 1987;**14**:183

[46] Hurt WG, Cooke CL, Jordan WP, Bullock JP, Rodriguez GE. Behçet's syndrome associated with pregnancy. Obstetrics and Gynecology. 1979;**53**:315

[47] Madkour M, Kudwah A. Behçet's disease. British Medical Journal.

1978;**2**:1786. DOI: 10.1136/bmj.2.6154.1786-a

[48] Farrag OA, Al-Suleiman SA, Bella H, Al-Omari H. Behçet disease in pregnancy. The Australian and New Zealand Journal of Obstetrics and Gynaecology. 1987;**27**:161-163. DOI: 10.1111/j.1479-828X.1987.tb00972.x

[49] Gürler A, Erdi H. The course of Behçet's disease in pregnancy. Turkiye Klinikleri Journal of Dermatology. 1995;**5**:125-128

[50] Kale A, Akyildiz L, Akdeniz N, Kale E. Pregnancy complicated by superior vena cava thrombosis and pulmonary embolism in a patient with Behçet disease and the use of heparin for treatment. Saudi Medical Journal. 2006;**27**:95-97

[51] Komaba H, Takeda Y, Fukagawa M. Extensive deep vein thrombosis in a postpartum woman with Behçet's disease associated with nephrotic syndrome. Kidney International. 2007;**71**:6. DOI: 10.1038/sj.ki.5001839

[52] Seyahi E, Yazıcı H. Pregnancy and Behçet's disease: Comment on the Article by Noel et al. Arthritis and Rheumatism. 2013;**65**(11):3007. DOI: 10.1002/art.38126

[53] Nadzi A, Sharma F, Jamshidi AR, Davachi F. Behçet's disease and pregnancy. Acta Medica Iranica. 2004;**42**:415-418

[54] Wilson WA, Gharavi AE, Koike T, Lockshin MD, Branch DW, Piette JC, et al. International consensus statement on preliminary classification criteria for definite antiphospholipid syndrome: Report of an international workshop. Arthritis and Rheumatism. 1999;**42**:1309-1311. DOI: 10.1002/1529-0131(199907)42:7<1309::AID-ANR1>3.0.CO;2-F

[55] Espinosa G, Cervera R, Reverter JC, Tassies D, Font J, Ingelmo M. Vascular involvement in Behçet's disease. The Israel Medical Association Journal. 2002;**4**:614-616. 29

[56] Krause I, Weinberger A. Vasculo-Behçet's disease. The Israel Medical Association Journal. 2002;**4**:636-637

[57] Diav-Citrin O, Shechtman S, Schwartz V, Avgil-Tsadok M, FinkelPekarsky V, Wajnberg R, et al. Pregnancy outcome after in utero exposure to colchicine. American Journal of Obstetrics and Gynecology. 2010;**203**:144.e1-144.e6. DOI: 10.1016/j.ajog.2010.02.063

[58] Berkenstadt M, Weisz B, Cuckle H, Di-Castro M, Guetta E, Barkai G. Chromosomal abnormalities and birth defects among couples with colchicine treated familial Mediterranean fever. American Journal of Obstetrics and Gynecology. 2005;**193**:1513-1516. DOI: 10.1016/j.ajog.2005.03.043

[59] Ahn JK, Lee YS, Jeon CH, Koh EM, Cha HS. Treatment of venous thrombosis associated with Behçet's disease: Immunosuppressive therapy alone versus immunosuppressive therapy plus anticoagulation. Clinical Rheumatology. 2008;**27**:201-205. DOI: 10.1007/s10067-007-0685-z

[60] Marchioni RM, Lichtenstein GR. Tumor necrosis factor-α inhibitor therapy and fetal risk: A systematic literature review. World Journal of Gastroenterology. 2013;**19**:2591-2602. DOI: 10.3748/wjg.v19.i17.2591

[61] Cheent K, Nolan J, Shariq S, Kiho L, Pal A, Arnold J. Case report: Fatal case of disseminated BCG infection in an infant born to a mother taking infliximab for Crohn's disease. Journal of Crohn's and Colitis. 2010;**4**:603-605. DOI: 10.1016/j.crohns.2010.05.001

[62] Djokanovic N, Klieger-Grossmann C, Pupco A, Koren G. Safety of

infliximab use during pregnancy. Reproductive Toxicology. 2011;**32**:93-97. DOI: 10.1016/j.reprotox.2011.05.009

[63] Alpsoy E. New evidence-based treatment approach in Behçet's disease. Pathology Research International. 2012;**2012**:871019. DOI: 10.1155/2012/871019